Moments of Rupture: The Importance of Affect in Education and Surgical

This book introduces the notion of affective thinking, which intersects the fields of education, critical humanities and healthcare.

Through practice-based pedagogic inquiry, it explores how a learner can experience moments of practice in which their established and familiar ways of thinking and knowing are ruptured. Employing a philosophical framework, grounded in theories of affect and related concepts, it examines how unanticipated events of practice impact professional beliefs, knowledge, skills and ethics. Drawing on the writings and theories of a select group of philosophers – Alfred North Whitehead, Michel Foucault, Gilbert Simondon, Gilles Deleuze and Brian Massumi – the author derives a novel paradigm in professional education, 'affective thinking', to describe the processes that initially occur when professionals first encounter an unexpected event of learning or practice. To illustrate this paradigm, the book draws on three sources of data: interviews with surgeons, training materials and clinical guidelines in medicine, and ethnographic accounts of clinical practice from the UK and USA. In doing so, the book explores ways of learning that are presently obscured by established discourses in pedagogy, education and professional practice.

The book will be of interest to those working in all aspects of healthcare, as well as students and scholars of the medical humanities and education.

A. O. Mahendran is a senior lecturer and consultant transplant surgeon at Queen Mary University/Barts and the Official name of university is Barts and the London School of Medicine and Dentistry, where she is also programme director for the MSc. in Physician Associate Studies. She undertook her specialist surgical training in London and New York and completed a PhD in education at Goldsmiths', University of London. She was the 2018 Winner of the (BERA) British Educational Research Association Doctoral Thesis Award.

Routledge Advances in the Medical Humanities

For more information about this series visit: www.routledge.com/Routledge-Advances-in-the-Medical-Humanities/book-series/RAMH

Moments of Rupture: The Importance of Affect in Medical Education and Surgical Training

Perspectives From Professional Learning and Philosophy

A. O. Mahendran

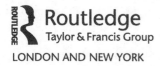
Routledge
Taylor & Francis Group

LONDON AND NEW YORK

First published 2020
by Routledge
4 Park Square, Milton Park, Abingdon, Oxon OX14 4RN
605 Third Avenue, New York, NY 10017

First issued in paperback 2023

Routledge is an imprint of the Taylor & Francis Group, an informa business

© 2020 A. O. Mahendran

British Library Cataloguing-in-Publication Data
A catalogue record for this book is available from the British Library

Library of Congress Cataloging-in-Publication Data
A catalog record for this book has been requested

ISBN: 978-1-03-257049-5 (pbk)
ISBN: 978-1-138-31757-4 (hbk)
ISBN: 978-0-429-45514-8 (ebk)

DOI: 10.4324/9780429455148

Typeset in Times New Roman
by Apex CoVantage, LLC

Publisher's Note
The publisher has gone to great lengths to ensure the quality of this reprint but
points out that some imperfections in the original copies may be apparent.

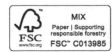

Printed in the United Kingdom
by Henry Ling Limited

Contents

Acknowledgements

This book has been many years in the making and traversed important experiences and milestones in my life – surgical trainee, budding educator, consultant surgeon, wife and mother. Therefore, I begin by offering special thanks to Amma and Appa, who have nourished me in all my adventures with deep affection and unconditional support. I am particularly grateful to my husband, Ludovic, who has sustained me through the trials of writing a book with his patience, love, devotion and enormous capacity to read and re-read whatever I put in front of him. Particular thanks to Jon Jezak for his support and skilled writer's eye.

I want to thank colleagues and friends who have read the chapters, made comments or suggestions or taken time to engage in thoughtful and useful conversations that have allowed me to improve or develop further some of the ideas. They are Dennis Atkinson, Henri Ghesquiere, Tony Brown, Roger Kneebone, Linda de Cossart, Della Fisher, Alex Moore, Kirsten Dalrymple, Valerie Farnsworth and Fiona O'Rourke. I am grateful to all my interviewees who participated in good faith and shared in honesty their experiences and thoughts. This feat is particularly impressive given their frequent fatigue and hectic schedules.

Some of the chapters benefited from presentations and seminars I gave over the previous years in which the ideas were discussed and debated. I thank the students and audience for their participation and contributions. Some of the stories and concepts discussed in this book have appeared in other articles over the years.

Finally, I am thankful to the Routledge team for being so patient and supportive.

Illustrations

Figures

Table

Part I

Context and Theory

1 Introduction

Encountering the messiness of life, learning and practice

A Stolen Harvest

We change into scrub suits, I glance at the white, hospital clock, 10.52pm. The night has yet to begin. The operating theatre is large, cold with a faint whiff of detergent. Vinny, the senior surgeon, vigorously scrubs his hands creating an impressive pink froth. As I dry my hands I think back to earlier in the evening and a fateful conversation with Mr. Carrick, my senior trainer.

"What are you up to this evening?" The tone was nonchalant, but the fixed look in his eyes conveyed a serious purpose. In turn, I faithfully reproduced the expected response, "Hmmmm, nothing important. How can I help Mr. Carrick?"

"We need an extra pair of hands on the organ retrieval tonight. . . . you haven't been on one before, have you . . .?"

Masked, gloved and gowned in sky blue robes, we perch on stools against the theatre door. I ask Vinny, "how many retrievals have you done?" His eyes betray the years of sleepless nights spent harvesting. An organ procurement or retrieval surgery is an operation in which a person who is dying gives prior consent to have their organs removed on death. These surgeries on the not-dead-yet are usually conducted in the unsocial, godless hours between night and twilight. The organs are then implanted in patients on waiting lists with liver, kidney or heart failure. It gives these human lives a second chance. Retrieval teams can travel far and wide to harvest organs. However, the destination always remains the same, a place between the portals of life and death.

I request that as both kidneys are to be retrieved, could I watch him remove the right kidney and then he supervise me with taking out the left? I reassert that he must let me do the procedure by myself; how else am I to learn? The transplant coordinator darts her head through the theatre door and sharply orders us, "the donor is here, everyone be quiet!" (The donor is the patient who has been diagnosed with brain death, kept alive by a heart and lung machine.) The whir of the patient trolley wheels can be heard in the distance, growing nearer with each microsecond. I can also hear a shuffle of feet – the donor is being brought to the theatre doors accompanied by a few members of the family and the nursing staff. Outside the theatre door lie the remaining vestiges of a human life in all its fading colours. Inside the theatre room lies the ultimate destiny of this human life – an offering of their tissues and organs.

Death cannot be coerced or hurried into a time of our choosing. Neither will it politely oblige or fall in line with our convenience. The living, however, are required to be punctual. A retrieval team must be ready to swing into action as soon as death has been pronounced. Our philosophy is, 'always early, but never late'. The breathing apparatus is stopped. The sound of the donor's family softly weeping and their heart wrenching sobs waft through what is supposed to be an impenetrable theatre door – a fierce barrier against the spread of infection and disease, but not, it seems, an impervious screen against the human condition. I feel anxious and uneasy, agitating in my gown. I was not prepared for this?! All that had been discussed was the placement of the incision, "from suprasternal notch to pubis," and "clamp the aorta, move with speed, quickly dissect those tissues, there's not much time to get those organs out . . . ." Instead, here I am occupying a limbo land – a place where life has been extinguished but death has not quite taken hold, just yet.

The Hindus believe that after the moment of death has passed, the soul of the deceased floats in the atmosphere, waiting for passage into the afterlife. It's a bit like occupying a seat in a waiting room, biding one's time. I've often wondered what the lingering spirit of a donor patient would make of my surgical handiwork. Would they peer over my shoulder and remark that my hands could be steadier, my dissection more precise and surely, I could work with more speed?! Would they 'tut-tut' resignedly or 'hmmmm' in approval? Would the surgery school report read, 'has real potential but must try harder!'

The doors swing open abruptly and the trolley is whisked in. The team turn their faces away. Too late. I see her face. Pale, puffy, swollen skin turgid from the weeks of medications and futile life-saving treatments. Brown, dishevelled hair, grey-blue eyes, dilated, staring into the blank air. I am rooted to the ground, stunned. Vinny seeing my distress, barks, "cover her face . . . Arundi, come over here and don't look . . ." He knows it is too late to warn me. She will now live in a piece of my brain that frequently wakes me up at night with thoughts and images of things I have seen and done. Another person to haunt my being. Her body is transferred and quickly prepared for surgery.

KW – Organ Donor	*Kimberley Walsh – Human Being*
32-year-old female non-heart beating donor. Cause of death; large cerebral haemorrhage following an RTA (road traffic accident). Hit by oncoming turning vehicle at 40mph. Past medical history: fit and well, D&C (dilatation and curettage) for a miscarriage two years ago. Non-smoker, social drinker. Cervical smear in November clear. Last urine output 72 mls/ hour, creatinine 93 mmol/l, blood pressure 110/72, not required inotropes. Registered organ donor. Family at first refused permission for donation to proceed.	*Kim is 32 next Wednesday. Lives in Crouch End opposite the clock tower with flat mates Kerry and Sunil. Mum and Dad still live in Bournemouth, brother Jo has also relocated to London. Kim has been dating Neil, whom she met at a friend's party three months ago. They were planning a week's break in Malaga at the end of September. Kim teaches year 12 at Cranford Secondary School. She loves cycling and running marathons, is a fully qualified diver. Knocked off her bike three weeks ago whilst cycling home from work.*

There is no time to dwell on those eyes. Brush it away. Bury it. But it remains, simmering beneath a veneer. Get on with the job. You have the living to contemplate now. Vinny grabs the knife from me. I have failed at my first organ procurement. The stealth with which he cuts and dissects the tissues is remarkable. He enters the abdominal cavity where the stash we have come for is being held. I watch, numb and paralysed. I had wanted to do this operation so much, but right now I have neither thoughts nor words that can articulate just how I feel at this moment. Later when we're finished, Vinny pats me on the back saying stiffly and somewhat awkwardly, "Uhh . . . don't worry . . . there'll be a next time . . . you just need to do more, that's all."

How do I make sense of this strange harvest? We are errant farmers, appearing in the night to steal and abscond with a harvest that we have neither sown nor cultivated to maturity. We were not present at the time of birth to thrill at the beautifully formed fingers and toes, to take pride when the first few words were uttered, to nurse knees grazed on the school playground or to pack a car full of things to be debunked at a university dorm. Instead, we are robber farmers from a limbo land. Reaping a harvest which is carefully and dutifully implanted in the battered landscape of another human being. This harvest, stolen in the night, can nourish a diseased body and provide hope where there was little to begin with. This is the lived reality of our task. But today, I'm not sure that I have what it takes to be a robber farmer. And I'm not sure that I want to be a robber farmer, anymore.

1.1 What is this book about? Who is it for?

This narrative of a young surgeon 'cutting her teeth' in transplant surgery is *my* story, illustrating how an encounter with the *reality* of surgical practice deeply *affected* me. In those early years, I would eagerly grab training opportunities like this one – participating in a procedure that junior trainees considered folklore, a surgery that was steeped in mystery and allure. That night, I had expected to operate and acquire a 'hands-on' experience of organ procurement, reinforcing my pre-procedure reading and technical discussions with senior colleagues. However, what I actually experienced at the surgery was profoundly unsettling and wholly unexpected. In addition, my supervisor, Vinny, had not anticipated my reaction either and later attempted to brush off the incident. Even after all these years I struggle to verbalise what it was that I actually *felt* in those *immediate moments of encounter* and why I was incapacitated, unable to make a skin incision. Over time, I have experienced other clinical events which in those immediate moments of encounter have disturbed, disrupted or slowed down my practice. All this is rather abstract and a challenge to put into words, but, more to the point, why does it even matter? It is precisely this issue of *mattering* that concerns me in this book. I suggest that how I immediately respond in this encounter with the deceased patient – what I describe as the *speechlessness of experience* – relates to my unconscious attempt to *grasp* the experience, to make sense of it, to begin to process it and create meaning. In those initial moments of encounter, an individual is confronted with the 'newness' of the experience, its unfamiliarity and strangeness, evoking non-conscious feelings that reflect how the encounter begins to matter to the person. This book attempts to articulate these emotional dimensions of clinical practice from the insider perspective.

Although the book is informed by research data gathered from the experiences and training practices of surgeons, a community I belong to and am very familiar with, it is written for healthcare professionals, medical/clinical educators as well practitioners and researchers who are interested in its main objective: an exploration of the *affective conditions* that emerge from disturbances in practice and their power to shape, construct and transform how professionals understand their practice and function within it.

In the narrative, the potent odours, the graphic images of flesh, the strange textures and life-altering events, elicit strong sensations and responses, triggering a *world of affects and senses* that constitute the reality of the encounter for the individual surgeon. Through these powerful affective experiences, an encounter with practice starts to become meaningful to the practitioner, taking on a significance for that individual and potentially leading to ontological and epistemological growth.

1.2   The theoretical struggle of this project: examining aspects of experience which are obscured

In situations similar to the opening narrative, it is not uncommon to dwell on moments of uncertainty which relate to the intensities of affect: *'What do I do here? How must I think or act? How do I carry on?'* On occasion, as described in the narrative, these emotional states can overwhelm one. However, a key feature of a clinician's practice is the ability to perform in uncertain or contingent environments in which events cannot be adequately prepared for in advance. A focus on the practical aspects of a task, such as concentrating on the steps of a procedure, can help a practitioner navigate the turbulence of the unanticipated affective state and avoid incapacitation. However, a singular pursuit of the technical steps to a task can also reduce the emerging affective components of the encounter to the category of 'inconvenient emotions'. The result is that affective behaviours are perceived as more of a hindrance to decisive action rather than a potential strategic tool in practice. But, as discussed in this book, the affective connections that emerge from unexpected clinical experiences can form important modes of learning and enquiry. These statements do not diminish or minimize the critical importance of learning practical skills, particularly in a craft specialty like Surgery. Instead, I argue for an approach that acknowledges the co-existing value of affective learning while recognizing its potential to extend existing pedagogic strategies in education and training.

To illustrate this argument, I use the example of how my practice as a trainer evolved and developed as a direct result of the narrated incident. I could empathise with and understand the educational difficulties that face trainees: predominantly, attempting to learn in unpredictable clinical situations, rich in affective consequences. I designed inductions and simple simulations to progressively immerse trainees in surgical practice. This included a formal initiation period to operative culture which involved exposing surgical trainees to empty operating theatres after hours, when no other staff were present. I anticipated, given my own experience as a new trainee many years ago, that in this new environment, a novice surgeon might develop affective responses on being introduced to aspects of surgery. The culture of the operating theatre is, amongst other things, fast paced, quick thinking, high stakes, unexpected, sexist, hierarchical, adrenaline dripping, all consuming, often joyous and sometimes devastating. A veritable fabric of affect can envelop and overwhelm a surgeon.

These initial student forays into surgical culture were designed to provide learning spaces for the trainee, so that the affective impact of clinical experiences could be facilitated, supported and *unpacked*. The latter refers to examining something of interest in detail in order to understand its nature. Such a process is important to make visible how affective responses modulate our ways of seeing, doing and understanding in clinical practice and learning. My aim was to help students recognise and reflect on their affective responses in comfortable, unpressured operative environments that permitted the development of individual awareness and personal strategies that would prove useful when forced to cope and learn with real events of actual surgical practice. What I have described is akin to the objectives of simulation training, a fast-developing area of skills acquisition in surgical education. However, my goal is separate to the objectives of standard simulation training. I seek to cultivate an affective awareness in professional (surgeon) training, which may have implications for both the technical and non-technical aspects of a student's ability.

How can one investigate the affective dimensions of clinical practice, a nebulous aspect of learning experiences? How can the implications of the affective dimension for learning, teaching and practice be demonstrated or understood? These questions reflect some of the challenges that this project attempts to meet.

No discussion of clinical experience is complete without recognising how professional regulations, systems of assessment and performance measurements impact and control the ways in which clinical practice is enacted. Therefore, the second aim of this book is to explore how these aspects of modern medicine, responsible for organising and regulating clinical learning and practice, control, enable or frustrate a clinician's ability to respond and react in appropriate ways. If it appears that this book is confirmation that I possess all the answers regarding the emotional character of learning and practice, please be forewarned that I do not! Instead, I attempt to instigate discussion about the affective nature of practice: what are its implications for the development of technical proficiency and clinical skill? How does it impact emerging professional identities? What is its role in shaping behaviours and attitudes in clinical practice? Readers are encouraged to engage critically with the ideas and concepts shared in these pages to compare my illustrations of theory with their own thoughts about and experiences of learning and professional practice.

1.3 What themes emerge from an affective exploration of clinical practice?

In writing this book I have attempted to move beyond the dominant discourses within medical education and clinical training, which focus on outcomes and assessment, to consider the power of learning encounters to precipitate new or modified ontological and epistemological states within an individual. In other words, what concerns me is how learners emerge from events of practice with *expanded capacities to think, see, understand and behave*. In this conception of pedagogy, prescribed and established pathways of learning and practice are relaxed in favour of exploring the conditions that emerge from actual events of learning and which contribute to the transformation of the practitioner. Here I turn to Tim Ingold (2015, p. 157) who has described pedagogic work as a *joining with* learners 'in an on-going exploration of what the possibilities and potentials of learning might be'. He advocates contemplating learning beyond the instructions of curriculum, learning objectives and outcomes and the scrutiny of assessment strategies. Thus, the main exploration of this book centres on *how* trainees learn rather than *what* trainees should learn (and the ways in which this assimilation of knowledge can be measured).

This investigation of *how* trainees learn is aligned with interrogating processes of *being and becoming* a surgeon/professional, which in the surgical education literature was emphasized by Linda de Cossart and Della Fisher in their critical publication *Cultivating a Thinking Surgeon* (2005). Such a pedagogic project intimately connects how something becomes significant to learners (i.e. how trainees learn) with their inherent abilities and condition (who they are, what beliefs they hold etc.) rather than conceiving trainees as empty vessels to be filled.

Here I outline the principal themes that emerge from the research conducted into this way of considering clinical learning encounters.

Ruptures in practice

The opening narrative and other stories contained in this book are illustrations of how a particular clinical *event* can function to *rupture* the standard practices of a professional. In these circumstances, 'event' is understood as something that *disturbs or punctures* established ways of thinking or acting. For example, the accepted practice at the organ procurement included a rapid and efficient surgical technique to carefully excise important organs for future transplantation. However, my encounter with the deceased organ donor was not consistent with the expected and approved ways of conducting oneself in this surgery. Standard practices are accepted as the 'norm' because they are historic ('this is how we've always done things') or aligned with the prevalent values of the age or the product of evidence-based research and therefore formally endorsed by the profession. I hasten to add that in making these statements I do not criticise the established skills, knowledge or decision-making processes that constitute the majority of safe and effective clinical practices. Instead, what I emphasise is the difficulty that arises when a clinician's conduct falls outside of these acceptable patterns of professional thought and behaviour. This is the power of the 'event', moments of clinical experience which *disrupt* standard practices. What can this disruption yield?

To explore this notion of event and its potential consequences I turn to Alain Badiou, a French philosopher: 'a truth is solely constituted by rupturing with the order which supports it, never as an effect of that order. I have named this type of rupture which opens up truths "the event"' (2005, p. 12). For Badiou an event has the potential to fracture the familiar and known, to disclose new or modified capacities to see, think, make and feel ('truths'). Therefore, a person can emerge from an event with heightened abilities and capacities to think and act in practice – qualities not present prior to the event. The challenge for trainers and educators is to develop pedagogic strategies that can recognise and facilitate the productive nature of ruptures to practice.

Coping and learning in the 'thisness' of practice

Surgeons and other healthcare professionals frequently grapple with the 'messy' reality of actual practice in an attempt to make sense of, learn from and negotiate the complexities of actual clinical experiences. In the narrative this is exemplified by how I stood in the operating theatre 'forced' to engage with the 'here-and-now' or 'thisness' of the experience. The notion of 'thisness' relates to being immersed in the ebb and flow of an encounter as it unfolds in uncertain and unforeseeable ways. It is a translation from Latin of the medieval scholastic philosophy, *'haecceities'*. At the organ procurement, the thisness of the encounter for me was constituted by the warmth radiating from a recently deceased corpse, the sight of a dilated pair of blue eyes sunken in a puffy pale face and the sounds of a family's heart-wrenching grief. The knowing that emerges from these unexpected encounters with real practice, powerful and enduring, is grounded in the *thisness* of the experience, whereas established bodies of knowledge, for example curriculum or clinical guidelines, represent forms of knowing that are abstracted from actual experiences of practice.

This leads me to the paradox of practice: reconciling what is taught and assimilated with what transpires when engaging with the realities of clinical experience. Negotiating this continual tension requires an awareness and appreciation of the *specific relations of practice* that constitute the different forms of knowing. Here I turn to Gilles Deleuze (2004), another French philosopher, and his work on 'transcendence' and 'immanence'. In simple terms, transcendence refers to established or fixed criteria that are used to judge something, for example, surgical training assessments (DOPS,[1] CBD[2]) used to evaluate a trainee's operative performance. In this example, what is examined is how closely a trainee meets the *transcendent* criteria of a particular assessment. In contrast, the notion of immanence concerns the relations that develop and emerge from within actual experiences of practice, which resonates with the thisness of a situation.

In medical education and clinical practice, transcendent categories of knowledge and skill are critical to the development of safe and competent practice. However, recognising the limits of these established forms of knowing are important, particularly when learning encounters arise that do not fit the specific parameters of the transcendent format, potentially foreclosing the development of new ways to learn, teach or practice. For example, at the procurement surgery, my inability to operate meant that I failed the technical task. Nonetheless, the event constituted a powerful learning encounter for me – I began to develop a new understanding of what it meant to be a transplant surgeon, an authentic perspective which brought home to me the challenges and complexities that would characterise my professional life.

Existing assessment structures cannot appropriately capture the lived reality of clinical experiences nor the dynamic and fluid nature of learning encounters. The incorporation and promotion of reflective practice in dealing with these complexities and challenges in clinical work has not proved as effective a strategy as was initially proposed (Boud and Walker 1998). I elaborate on this in further chapters.

Becoming undone: how something matters to an individual

At the procurement surgery when I accidentally catch sight of the patient's face, it precipitates a *becoming undone* for me. In these moments of uncertainty, *I risk myself* attempting to grasp this strange experience in an effort to cope with and make sense of it. The 'risk' relates to being forced to respond, act and think in ways that fracture the security of established knowledge and methods. This notion of 'becoming undone', taken from Judith Butler's work (2005), concerns how a learner becomes uncertain, destabilised or *undone* when forced to challenge the established knowledge and practices in an attempt to grasp the potential of the *unknown*. The unknown *is not* a reference to the finite knowledge and skills contained in surgical textbooks and curriculae (transcendent frameworks) which are taught on training programmes. Rather, the unknown represents *that-which-is-yet-to-be*, modes of learning and their outcomes that are yet to emerge but which constitute how an encounter with practice comes to matter, attains relevance and significance for that particular subject.

As such, engaging with the unknown can lead to developing knowledge, skills and understanding that exceed what the practitioner has achieved up to this point in their practice. The concept of that-which-is-yet-to-be is explored in later chapters through the work of Gilles Deleuze. These concepts are useful when considering how to reconfigure learning and teaching in clinical environments to include *a trainee's attempts to grasp the unknown* and a trainer's efforts to *draw alongside* that complex experience. The notion of 'drawing alongside' a learner relates to the trainer/educator attempts to connect with the changes and potentials that are brought about my new experiences in order to understand how that aspect of practice matters for the learner. In this paradigm of medical education, pedagogic work is viewed as a 'risky' *adventure* where the learning outcomes are not always predictable, clear or visible and may not coincide with the formal teaching objectives or assessment criteria.

To attempt this requires a softening of the transcendent parameters of practice that currently frame clinical events to consider more carefully the emerging modes of becoming. Gert Biesta (2006, 2010; Bingham and Biesta 2010) has written extensively on these ideas, influenced by the writings of Jacques Ranciere. He examines how 'the learner', 'the student' and the different ways in which learners learn are conceived. In brief, he argues that the term 'learner' is constructed through the notion of 'lack' because the student moves away from a state of 'not knowing' through the intervention of a teacher. However, a teacher's instruction or explanation must *matter* to the student in order for that learning encounter to be potentially transformative, leading to modified capacities to understand, learn or do. Therefore, *that-which-is-yet-to-be* is not a state of 'lack' but rather an attempt to become undone, to grasp the uncertain substance of the learning encounter, which can compel expanded capacities to think and act.

The speechlessness of experience: encounters with affect

The reader may have noticed by now that the notion of 'encounter' is a core and pervading motif of this book. I use 'encounter' to describe how an individual initially *takes account of something*, how she perceives or grasps an object, a person or situation for example. In other words, how is this *something* initially experienced? This application of encounter resonates with Alfred North Whitehead's (1929) concept of 'prehension', which relates to how an individual comes to *know* something through language or the senses in ways that make a difference to her. To illustrate this, I return to how I initially *prehended* the event of organ procurement: through the colours and odours of the operating theatre, the images and sounds of death and dying. This pressing reality, both inescapable and unanticipated, is rooted in the *speechlessness of experience* – I am slowed down and suspended in a dimension that *precedes* consciousness, where cognitive processes are yet to emerge and organise the experience through language, logic and reflection. The condition of 'speechlessness' also draws attention to how moments of uncertainty or unfamiliarity can precipitate immediate *affective states* of being, which are non-conscious and therefore difficult to articulate even months and years after the encounter has come to pass. However, through these initial affective relations, the subject encounters practice in ways that are pre-cognitive and non-rational. This is the *affective dimension* of experience through which the subject first comes to *know* the event of practice. It signifies how that encounter with practice starts to attain a *relevance* for her.

The forms of knowing that arise from these *local flows of experience* represent 'affective thinking', which as I discuss later in this book impact the development of learners' technical proficiency, relationships in the workplace as well as emerging identities and attitudes to professional practice. These notions of learning do not diminish the importance of established theories of learning, bodies of knowledge and skill or current modes of assessment in medical education and clinical training (*transcendent* frameworks of practice). Instead, I query how to extend paradigms in clinical education and training to support and facilitate the novel intensities and ideas that emerge from unanticipated experiences of practice.

The speechlessness of experience exceeds those arguments that solely attribute my muteness and paralysis to a lack of exposure to this type of surgery, the inexperience typical of a novice surgeon. As Vinny advises me in the story, the antidote is to do more! Whilst I acknowledge that a lack of exposure to procedures or other practices can trigger features of shock, to conclude that my responses are largely due to inexperience is to neglect to acknowledge the affective states that emerge from encounters with practice and their implications for learning and coping in contingent practice.

Why is this relevant to practitioners and educators engaged in the many healthcare professions? The contingency of clinical practice has two major applications for surgical education. First, it requires surgeons to make decisions in unfamiliar situations, trying to find a way forward to meet the needs of the patient. An awareness of the affective dimension is particularly important when addressing the uncertainty of clinical situations. It engenders an improved self-awareness in practice as the learner recognizes how thoughts and actions are precipitated or influenced. This also has important implications for how policy is constructed in healthcare, bringing to attention the ways in which the affective nature of behaviour can impact policy enactment.

Second, affective modes of experiencing may contribute to the emergence of qualities in surgical trainees which are neither visible nor tangible through the conventional training assessment – for example, the assessment of clinical decision making through a learner's ability to 'talk through' the steps of their process. This relies on a linguistic grammar to demonstrate assimilation of knowledge and an ability to rationalize. The difficulty arises when this assessment format is developed around a learner's language ability. This may mean that what is examined is not the skill of decision making but rather the ability to communicate one's thoughts. As a consequence, the affective aspects of decision making become invisible and are not considered as relevant or valuable by existing pedagogic discourses.

The notion of affect delineates the feelings and emotions that arise out of the encounters and events that we experience. These *affectations* push and pull us in various directions, which in turn impact our thoughts, actions and decision-making processes. Our affective states control and modulate how we perceive and respond to unfolding events thus precipitating onto-epistemological potentials for the individual. Recognising and understanding the nature of affect in learning and practice can help support and foster more effective learners as well as thoughtful, confident practitioners.

Negotiating established clinical guidance and recommended practice: the impact of hylomorphism

We live at a time of rapid social changes, where numerous policy initiatives drive societal efforts to structure, streamline and regulate professional education. These attempts to professionalise education seek to ensure that learners are accountable, transparent and competent. But have these systemic changes equipped learners and practitioners to better cope and manage the complexities that arise from the inherent uncertainty of actual practice? I explore these questions by comparing and contrasting the official guidelines for practice with actual experiences of everyday practice. What emerges from this analysis is that efforts to structure the chaos of 'real' practice and guarantee specific learning outcomes have led to established categories of what is deemed appropriate and relevant medical knowledge or skill being applied to encounters of practice (Law and Mol 2002; Greenhalgh 2013, 2014). Examples include the development of protocols, clinical pathways and algorithms, which collectively constitute formal clinical epistemologies to combat the uncertainty of medical practice and to prioritise the safety of the patient (Engebretsen et al. 2016). Earlier I described these forms of knowledge and skill as transcendent frameworks. The application of these transcendent forms to clinical practice functions to generate order and organisation to the chaos of experience.

To critically examine and better understand the implications of this approach to practice, I have drawn on the notion of *hylomorphism* as discussed by Aristotle in his ancient Greek writings. In essence, Aristotle observed that for an object to exist, to be perceptible or tangible, it must have a recognisable shape, structure or discernible form. He provides the example of marshy clay amorphous till moulded into a recognisable structure: a brick. I suggest that protocols, pathways, algorithms and assessment criteria represent hylomorphic structures – they attempt to organize the uncertainty of clinical practice into ordered and recognizable frameworks. After all, doctors must be able to act decisively, effectively and safely when caring for sick patients in risky and unpredictable situations.

The difficulty arises when learning encounters, which by nature are fluid and dynamic, are 'forced' into predefined categories of performance. This has the effect of organising the learning experience into something that can be easily analysed and assessed using current techniques. These educational strategies (unintentionally) homogenise learning encounters, by applying common principles derived from approved knowledge and practices. This approach removes potential opportunities to understand an *individual* experience of practice as it emerges from and relates to that particular learner.

Hylomorphic frameworks can appear to be rigorous or discriminatory in terms of how they identify and prioritise a learner's abilities. However, what they actually assess is how closely a trainee meets pre-identified criteria and whether that trainee's skill set is visible or demonstrable. In other words, what is not being assessed is the learner's inherent capacities, that is their intrinsic talents and skills, which may or may not fall within the boundaries of the hylomorphic assessment format.

1.4   How are the themes, arguments and research evidence structured?

This book is written as a journey through practice, exploring aspects of learning and teaching that arise when dealing with the uncertain nature of clinical environments and medical practice. There is a short introductory story to each chapter which is intended to engage the reader with the subject matter by firmly establishing the themes of the chapter and providing a trigger for the reader to develop questions and thoughts before proceeding to the main discussions and critiques. Some of the clinical stories are taken from my 15 years of surgical practice, whilst the remaining narratives are derived from the experiences of the research cohort of surgeons. It is not of concern to me in this book to discuss or debate the merits and challenges of narrative ethnography. This subject area is well investigated and written about in other distinguished works by fellow authors.

Chapter 2 builds on the introduction to affect by fleshing out this topic through a critical discussion of relevant philosophical theories. Do not despair, however, as the theories are made very simple through an application of common clinical scenarios. In particular, the difference between emotion and affect is established, as is how I use the concept of 'affect' in this book. Affect (theory) is explained as a phenomenon beyond the ways in which it is currently used by the medical/ clinical curriculum through descriptors such as the 'affective domain' and 'affective behaviours'.

Chapter 3 consolidates the theoretical arguments of this book by establishing an alternative yet complementary framework to traditional forms of learning and teaching – *pedagogies of encounter*. This conceptual framework recognises and accommodates the *singular nature of experiencing*, prioritising *how something matters* for the learner in that particular experience of practice. In practical terms, it is a call to address and explore the relations that constitute this 'how': how does the learner *encounter* the thisness of practice? What inherent abilities does the learner possess, which may not be identified by transcendent frameworks of practice (such as assessments)?

I recommend that Chapter 4 and 5 are read together, as they collectively provide an examination and discussion about how notions of Care in clinical practice are constructed, legitimised and enacted. The objective is to explore the differences between how care is developed and treated as a major concept within medical texts and clinical guidelines versus how to give appropriate care in unanticipated or unpredictable clinical situations.

Similarly, Chapters 6, 7 and 8 form a trilogy that explores how affective conditions of practice affect how surgeons experience clinical practice and how this is implicated in the ways in which professional identities are constructed. Chapter 6 examines the nature of these surgeon subjectivities through two interviews – one with a surgeon and one with a surgical educator. Chapter 7 explores how trainees are represented ('pedagogised') in training materials such as curriculum and assessment documents to identify how closely professional documents reflect the realities of practice which trainees must engage with.

Chapter 8 investigates how structures put in place to ensure the design and delivery of medical care (health policy, out-of-hours service provision) impact the affective responses of surgeons attempting to cope and learn in uncertain clinical encounters.

The final chapter, Chapter 9, brings together the ideas from the prior chapters to make suggestions for the development of future pedagogic strategies and practice.

1.5   Where does the data come from? How is it analysed?

I collected data from three sources, auto-ethnographic accounts of surgical training, surgeon interviews and a selection of training materials and professional handbooks that pertain to surgical practice as well clinical practice in general.

Over a decade spent in training I journaled my experiences of negotiating the challenges of training programmes first in the UK and then the USA. These biographical accounts illustrated how I was *affected* by my daily practice and how this effected the ways in which I constructed my ideas, behaviours and beliefs in practice. Similarly, in the interviews I conducted with surgeons, I encouraged them to recount stories of practice where an encounter with a clinical event had gone on to transform the way in which that particular surgeon conceptualised her practice. I believe that this emphasis on biographical accounts of practice prioritised my interest in the affective nature of experience and learning over a generic inquiry about professional attitudes and behaviours.

I have included excerpts from five interviews with surgeons – a mix of newly appointed consultants and senior trainees nearing completion of training – and one interview with an educator from the Royal College of Surgeons of England. I have anonymised all my interviewees, a necessary action given their honest responses and the sensitivity of the information they communicated. Where necessary I have altered the clinical details of patients and sometimes invented conditions to maintain confidentiality.

Readers may query why I chose this particular group of surgeons to interview – why not question more junior trainees or more senior surgeons? To which the simple answer is that of the many surgeons I contacted and ended up interviewing, this particular cohort, unlinked in terms of geography and speciality, were either available or made themselves available for interview. They took the time to listen to my repeated questions and answer as candidly as possible, never fatiguing or growing bored! The veracity of their answers does not concern me. I am not interested in proving whether or not their accounts accurately reflect what happened in factual terms. What interests me and what I prioritise in these pages is how they were impacted by their experiences and how they remember the incidents – it is the *nature of the experience* that concerns me. I electronically recorded all the discussions and made transcripts which accompanied my field notes from the interviews.

The training materials I chose to examine included the intercollegiate surgical curriculum for general surgery, a sample of work-based assessment tools as well as professional handbooks such as *Good Surgical Practice* (2014) and the GMC publication *Good Medical Practice* (2013) and relevant policy documents authorised by the Department of Health. All these materials were analysed using a theoretical framework which I set out in Chapters 2 and 3.

Examining the emotional dimension of practice is to engage with the *messiness of actual experiences* of learning and practice. Therefore, finding a theoretical approach that could accommodate the *multiple realities* embedded within encounters of practice was important to me. I returned to my ethnographic accounts of surgical practice where I had documented clinical events that illustrated themes such as providing care in complex environments, negotiating uncertainty in practice, navigating emotions in clinical contexts and attempting to learn clinical skills in difficult medical scenarios. I found that these themes were useful in guiding my reading of theoretical texts and through this endeavour I discovered that works of philosophy and their accompanying discourses were well suited to helping me unpack the intricacies and complexities of experiencing within clinical environments. The philosophers I have explored are either understudied or novel to medical education – Alfred North Whitehead, Alain Badiou, Gilbert Simondon, Gilles Deleuze and Brian Massumi – to name the principal theorists I turn to. I hope that their inclusion in directing the emerging discussions on 'experiencing' and 'affect' make a critical contribution to the existing research literature and debate on how emotions can modulate and influence the development of professional ways of seeing, thinking, understanding and acting.

1.6   Concluding remarks

I am particularly concerned with how the uncertain conditions of clinical practice are initially *affectively encountered* – what happens in those *moments of rupture*? Whilst this question can be examined from the perspective of a number of other disciplines and interests, I have sought a philosophical inquiry to guide this investigation as this approach resonates with my main objective – attempting to understand how something in practice comes to *matter* to a learner/professional. It is not my intention to provide a complete and authoritative book on emotion in clinical practice. Instead, I hope that through these stories of practice, readers will engage with how the theory can be used to make sense of similar experiences and take away some useful ideas, arguments and conclusions that may contribute to an enhanced understanding of learners and learning and their own encounters with professional practice.

Notes

1   Direct Observation of Procedural Skill.
2   Case-Based Discussion.

References

Badiou, A. (2005). *Handbook of Inaesthetics*. Stanford: Stanford University Press.

Biesta, G. (2006). *Beyond Learning; Democratic Education for a Human Future*. Boulder: Paradigm.

Biesta, G. (2010). "Learner, Student, Speaker: Why It Matters How We Call Those We Teach." *Educational Philosophy and Theory*, 42: 5–6.

Bingham, C., and Biesta, G. (2010). *Jacques Ranciere: Education, Truth Emancipation*. London and New York: Continuum.

Boud, D., and Walker, D. (1998). "Promoting Reflection in Professional Courses: The Challenge of Context." *Studies in Higher Education*, 23: 191–206.

Butler, J. (2005). *Giving an Account of Oneself*. Fordham University Press.

DeCossart, L., and Fish, D. (2005). *Cultivating a Thinking Surgeon: New Perspectives on Clinical Teaching*. TFM Publishing Ltd.

Deleuze, G. (2004). *Difference and Repetition*. London and New York: Continuum.

Engebretsen, E., Heggen, K., et al. (2016). "Uncertainty and Objectivity in Clinical Decision Making: A Clinical Case in Emergency Medicine." *Medicine, Health Care and Philosophy*. doi:10.1007/s11019-016-9714-5.

Greenhalgh, T. (2013). "Uncertain and Clinical Method." In Somers, L., and Launer, J. (Eds)., *Clinical Uncertainty in Primary Care: The Challenge of Collaborative Engagement*. New York: Springer.

Greenhalgh, T. (2014). "Evidence-Based Medicine: A Movement in Crises?" *British Medical Journal*, 348: g3725.

Ingold, T. (2015). The life of lines. London/New York: Routledge.

Law, J., and Mol, A. (2002). *Complexities: Social Studies of Knowledge and Practice*. Duke University Press.

Whitehead, A. N. (1929). *Process and Reality*. New York: The Free Press.

2 The Nature of Affect
a philosophical approach

.

This chapter and the next lay the theoretical framework for an exploration and analysis of how events of learning and practice are immediately experienced in clinical environs. In this chapter, the emotional complexities of professional life are examined through philosophical concepts that describe and explain the *affective flows of experience*. Now I am only too aware of how the phrase 'philosophical theory' can conjure images of dreary work grappling with dense text and abstract ideas with little practical advantage! With this in mind, the discussions on affect are presented in each section with a quick and easy summary of a particular idea followed by a more in-depth explanation for those readers inclined to read further.

I begin this chapter with a short story that describes my personal encounter with Mr. Martino, a patient who undergoes a serious medical complication when his body rejects his new liver transplant. Though I am familiar with the clinical features and management of acute organ rejection, I am wholly unprepared for Mr. Martino's reaction to his devastating new reality. This encounter informs the subject matter of this chapter, demonstrating the affective nature of clinical encounters and their power to moderate and influence ways of thinking, seeing, understanding, doing and learning in practice.

The narrative descriptions of my feelings, thoughts and behaviours may be construed as overly emotional, self-piteous, lacking in the appropriate detachment and objectivity expected of a professional, or simply viewed as an example of unprofessional conduct. Whilst all these criticisms may be accurate and fair, I included this auto-ethnographic account to illustrate the emotionally charged nature of many encounters with practice.

Such experiences of practice, constituted by difficult and challenging patient-doctor interactions in combination with heart-wrenching personal tragedy, often yield no obvious or easy solutions, such that there may be no 'right way' to act, although established codes of conduct can present practice in simplistic ways. In such situations, the *ethics of care* is imagined beyond notions of morality and professional codes of behaviour. It is an ethics relative to how one responds and emerges in the 'thisness' of the clinical encounter and all the inherent uncertainty that *affects* the thoughts, speech or actions that arise from the experience.

Crème Brûlée

"So . . . what d'you wanna do? I mean if *you* wanna talk to him, that's fine but I'm tellin' you, he's not listening and he's not gonna change his mind." She looks at me, expectant, twiddling the end of a twist of hair. It was her way of throwing down the gauntlet, her way of saying the unsaid; "if you think you can do better, go right ahead . . .". 'OK, Mary Ellen', I say. I am exhausted after spending the last 13 hours upright in a cold operating theatre, tackling what was supposed to have been a routine liver transplant. But the surgery turned out to be anything but routine.

I knock gingerly on the door of patient room 10. There is no answer. I knock again. Maybe he's asleep or in the bathroom, I reason. Or, maybe he's sitting in his bed, awake and he doesn't want to hear. I walk in slowly. "Mr. Martino, good morning. I just finished a surgery and thought I'd pop in and see how you are." Not quite the truth, but it will do. He does not meet my eyes, instead he stares out through the window, motionless. It is then that I notice sitting in the shadows at the back of the room, his wife and son. "Oh, I'm sorry, I didn't realise you had family here," (I nod my head at the family). "Well, good. Perhaps we can all have a chat together and see what we can do to get you stronger again." I try not to sound too chirpy: too much is always a step too far. The wife and son get up and move their chairs closer to Mr. Martino's bed, so that we are all now facing him. A jury sitting in judgement.

"I hear you won't eat anything. The nurses tell me that you haven't eaten in two days." I present the facts. "In fact, they say that you refuse all food, even the delicious food that Mrs. Martino brings in for you." I have upped the stakes and briefly glance at her, smiling weakly in a poor recognition of her efforts. Mrs. Martino however, is quietly sobbing. "He says this was a mistake," Luke, their son, suddenly interjects. He sounds worn and exasperated, motioning with his arms. "He says, that he knows this transplant has failed because he feels worse now than he did before the operation! He says he knows he's dying this time . . . no-one can save him." The opening statements have been made.

Mr. Martino remains still, his gaze fixed on the view out of the window. From the corner of my eye, I catch sight of the clock: 9.15am. The next patient for surgery would have been escorted to the operating suite by now (Grace Matthews, kidney transplant, right side). She's probably waiting for me in the anaesthetic room. In fact, the whole theatre team is most likely waiting for me and agitating as it becomes evident that my 'no-show' means the surgery is being delayed. Yet again. "OK," I sigh, put my hand in my pocket and switch off my phone. I walk over to the mobile table which is piled high with an incredible assortment of food, all cooked lovingly and patiently by Mrs. Martino.

I pick out a small glass dish containing a wonderfully aromatic crème brûlée, the vanilla and cinnamon are heavenly. I think back to three months ago when Julian Martino walked onto this same ward: disbelief, trepidation, wonder at the prospect of an impending liver transplant. Since then, one complication after another has weakened him and made his 'new' liver a hostile implant. He is presently in a state of acute organ rejection. For the second time in 12 weeks. The effects are florid and pernicious. A strong cocktail of anti-rejection drugs has eaten away at his tissues and destroyed his innate defences against disease. I perch on the edge of his bed, teetering on a precipice holding only dessert.

"I'm not going to lie to you and promise that everything will be better, that what you're going through now is temporary . . . not, because it isn't . . . but because I just don't know. When I told you that this liver transplant would mean a new life, a new beginning for you and your family, I truly believed it. Yes, I've seen things . . . bad things that happen when transplants go wrong, but that day when I came to talk to you here on the ward, I truly . . . in my heart . . . never thought that those bad things would happen to you, because you and the new liver seemed perfect for each other! It seemed like the chances of things not working out were so, so small." I continue to talk, slowly, the fatigue like a sponge in my brain, sucking up thoughts and words.

Normally I would have rehearsed this conversation mentally as I walked to his room, however, at this moment I am tired, hungry (damn this brûlée!) and irritated at the thought of the theatre staff waiting for me downstairs, most likely cursing me as they repeatedly reach my voicemail ("why the hell is her phone switched off?! Doesn't she know there's another case on the table!"). But mostly I am tired. Tired of offering explanations that are always inadequate because the promise of something better never quite materialises. Tired of the heroic efforts that fall short of finding a permanent solution to the disappointment and devastation of the few failed transplant lives. Tired, tired.

I twist and turn the spoon in my hand, a scalpel readying to slice the brûlée. Mr. Martino has not flinched once in the ten minutes I've been in the room. He continues to stare blankly out of the window, oblivious to my words, indifferent to my presence. He gives me nothing. I dig into the brûlée and scoop up a sliver of creamy flesh.

"I . . . if you don't eat, then what you're telling me, what you're telling the world is, 'I want to die' . . . because if you don't eat then that's what happens . . . you die, whether you've got a transplant inside you or not. And that's just not fair . . . it's not fair to them" (I point to his wife and son) "because all they want is to take you home, healthy and possibly even happy . . . and you know what sir? It's not fair to me . . . because that means I did a bad thing when I put that liver inside you . . . it means I did something to harm you . . . I hurt you in ways that I could never have imagined . . . and I am so so sorry because I can't undo it, I can't take out that liver, that thing that has poisoned you, because I have nothing to replace it with, absolutely nothing."

I can feel the tears welling in my eyes. "So, you can refuse all this glorious food cooked with so much love and hope because you've clearly given up on hope and you've clearly given up on me" (my voice starts to falter, I want to curl up at the foot of his bed and sleep and sleep. And forget). "I am so sorry. You will never know how sorry I am . . . you see I have nothing left to give you right now, not a thing . . . except . . . except this bloody amazing creme brûlée that I didn't even make for you . . . that's how lost I am with you." Julian Martino turns his impenetrable gaze to the creme brûlée, never once meeting my eyes. Without a word, he takes the spoon from my fingers and puts it to his lips. He chews slowly on the sweet flesh. Languid and methodical, he scoops out the contents of the dish all the while fixing his gaze out of the window.

There is no sign of whether he is enjoying it or not, in fact I think he eats not to taste.

I think he eats not because my words have resonated.

I think he eats not because hope has miraculously suffused his tissues.

At this moment in time, I think he eats to lighten my load.

I think he eats because he pities me.

I think he eats so that I may have hope again.

Whatever the reason, I gobble it up.

2.1   The emotional complexities of practice

Loss and *feeling* lost are dominant emotions that emerge from the affective forces that form and develop in this encounter. The atmosphere in the patient room is heavy with disease, morbidity and despair. Jeff Martino is bewildered and exasperated at this latest turn of events and even furious at his inability to control what is happening to his body and his health. Every day, treatments are administered, and promises are made by well-intentioned staff who are either unwilling to accept the serious consequences of the clinical problem or perhaps too cowardly to face the patient with the truth.

Mr. Martino retreats from the clinical plan. He withdraws from human relationships and any attempts to nourish his battered body. His disengagement may represent his effort to feel empowered again, to take back control of his life from the medical staff and seemingly futile treatments. Or it may be a sign of his deep despair and profound emotional pain. Add to this mix the desperation of his family and their attempts to support and lavish him with an abundance of food and attention. Mr. Martino's frightening and overwhelming experience, all too common, illustrate the strong motivations and important concerns that spearheaded the person-centred care (PCC) movement (Epstein and Street 2011; Coulter and Collins 2011). There are different frameworks for PCC, but the goal is the same – to share power and responsibility with patients within the therapeutic relationship so that the patient's needs and choices drive the care they receive (Harding et al. 2015; Hawkes 2015).

Then there is the weary surgeon, physically exhausted and emotionally drained by the endless demands of her clinical practice. My field notes from the day report my sense of feeling engulfed from the minute I stepped into Mr. Martino's room. I was overwhelmed by feelings of deep guilt, an inescapable sense of failing this patient – a man who had entrusted me with his health and life. Instead I was presiding over the erosion of his personhood. Sitting in that room, all of my perceived failures in practice returned to haunt me.

This narrative emphasises how the struggles of the past, the agonies of the present and the unforeseen events of the future can form undercurrents within any experience of professional practice, making it difficult to predict how one may *affect* an event, and in turn *be affected by* it.

2.2   The treatment of emotions in medical education research literature

Emotion and medical ability have long been seen as opposing forces in practice (Lief and Fox 1963; Dornan et al. 2015; MacLeod 2011). The display of emotion, associated with a caring, empathic identity, is at odds with the dispassionate approach seen as a precursor to clinical competence and equated with effective and successful professional practice. I remember being advised as a surgical trainee that emotionally tough and challenging practice would 'put hairs on your chest, just what you need!' The tendency to forge clinical expertise in the image of stereotyped masculine behaviours or what amounts to qualities of 'non-emotion' is based on traditional notions of professional resilience in medical practice which still persist today: emotional blunting, alongside detached and objective applications of science.

Such conceptions are supported by Shapiro's research (2011), which concluded that passage through medical training desensitised students to the effects of emotions. This is necessarily at odds with attempts to nurture emotionally sensitive clinicians who are better placed to provide person-centred care. However, a growing body of research has emerged in recent years advocating for the role of emotions in clinical learning and in the processes of being and becoming a doctor (Immordino-Yang and Damasio 2007; McConnell and Eva 2012). Nancy McNaughton (2013) examined discourses of emotion in medical education and identified three major conceptualisations of emotion: emotion as a consequence of a biological process, emotion as clinical competence to be demonstrated in specific skills and abilities and, finally, the sociocultural constructions of emotion derived from the humanities and social sciences.

Emotions are demonstrated to affect how information is assimilated, retrieved, interpreted and acted on (Blanchette and Richards 2010; Izard 2009). Emotions are not only implicated in student motivation to learn, but also in how we learn (Schutz and Pekrun 2007). However, the findings of these and other studies are in contrast to the prevalent practice whereby learners in medical fields tend to disregard or suppress their emotional thoughts and ideas for historic reasons, as well as for issues of convenience. The fast-paced, over-burdened healthcare environments have neither the capacity nor compulsion to support and 'work through' the emotional responses generated by challenging clinical practice.

Despite this, there is increasing interest and research in professional resilience and how to develop and implement strategies that promote and support clinicians confronted with the multiple stressors and high emotional labours associated with 21st-century clinical practice (McAllister and McKinnon 2009; Howe et al. 2012; Farquhar et al. 2018). Attending to emotional states goes beyond a concern for learner wellbeing, encompassing an appreciation and understanding of how practice comes to matter to an individual and the heightened capacities that can emerge when engaging with such clinical encounters.

2.2   What is 'affect'?

I have used 'affect' prodigiously without discussing *how* I am using it or *what* I mean by the term. My initial expectation was that the reader would appropriately infer from the content what I meant by 'affect'. In contrast, my actual experience of discussing this subject matter in seminars and conferences revealed just how unwise an assumption that would be. I am frequently asked to qualify what I mean as most participants understand 'affect' as a synonym for 'emotion' or 'feeling' and use the terms interchangeably.

Anthony Artino and Laura Naismith (2015) have commented on this 'long history of definitional disorder' (p. 140) in medical education research, which surrounds studies on emotion. They have attributed this situation in part to a consequence of the different research paradigms and scholarly work employed to investigate emotions in practice. Artino and Naismith define emotion as 'a psycho-physiological change that is short-lived, intense and specific to a personally meaningful stimulus' (ibid., p. 140). For example, I recall feeling embarrassment and shame after the organ procurement event when I failed to operate in a public setting. Emotions are therefore personal experiences, projections of feelings which emanate from our previous experiences and our memories of them. As such they are biographical and socially constructed.

Affect on the other hand is open to many interpretations. From Sigmund Freud (Breuer and Freud 2001) to Antonio Damasio (2000), the treatment of affect and its applications in the human being vary. In the spheres of neuroscience, biology, cognitive psychology, sociology, philosophy, media, film and gender studies and ethnography, affect has come to adopt many different meanings and connotations and is used differently by each discipline. An example is how Silvan Tompkins and Paul Ekman (Ekman 2007) conceptualised affective processes as independent of intention and meaning, while Sigmund Freud considered affects (he used 'affect' and 'emotion' interchangeably) as embodied, intentional states governed by beliefs, cognition and desires.

Within medical education as well as other healthcare professions such as nursing, the affective domain of practice is one of the three domains in Blooms Taxonomy, the other two being cognitive and psychomotor. The affective domain (Krathwohl et al. 1973) includes feelings, values, appreciation, enthusiasms, motivation and attitudes. It involves coping with and managing feelings, emotions, mindsets and values, nurturing desirable attitudes – reassuring patients, cultivating empathy and trust, demonstrating respect of colleagues and engaging in ethical practice. Attending to these aspects of the emotional dimension of practice is linked with enhancing the caring side of doctors both in terms of patient management and interactions with team members.

What ideas have influenced how I develop and use the notion of affect?

My interest in affect stems from my initial research efforts which explore events of experience and the *presentational immediacies of experience*. That is, I am interested in conceptual frameworks that help interrogate what happens in those *instantaneous moments of encounter*, when we are confronted by something that is unfamiliar and unknown in which we are yet to recognise the emotional content of the experience and organise it along familiar categories of reason and logic. In those immediate moments of encounter, there is but the 'affective hit' (Massumi 2008). It is this phenomenon, which is further elaborated on later, that forms the central exploration of this book.

I have explored research theories and philosophical writings that construct affect in these terms: *unconsciously experienced forces that arise from and within our continuous encounters of the world, exceeding the emergence of feelings and emotion.*

Affect remains intimately connected to the expression of feelings and emotions, as it *drives* us to think, feel, act and emote.

Kathleen Stewart, a cultural anthropologist and leading affect theorist explains the different ways in which affect can be experienced:

> they (affects) happen in impulses, sensations, expectations, daydreams, encounters, and habits of relating, in strategies and their failures, in forms of persuasion, contagion, and compulsion, modes of attention, attachment, and agency, and in public and social worlds of all kinds *that catch people up in something that feels like something.*
>
> (2007, pp. 1–2, original emphasis)

This notion of affect as 'something' that moves or impels us in our ordinary everyday lives as well as in exceptional circumstances (for example my experience at the organ procurement) has been similarly characterised by others as 'inclinations' (Leibniz 2008), 'drives' (Nietzsche 1982), 'intensities' and 'desires' (Deleuze and Guattari 1977) and 'thinking feeling' (Massumi 2008).

These descriptive terms share a common thread, that affect is *imperceptible*, because it arises prior to a conscious awareness of the phenomenon, nevertheless it is perceived or *felt* by virtue of the effects it exerts. For example, at the organ procurement surgery described in the introductory chapter, the powerful affective forces evolving from the encounter rendered me mute and physically incapacitated in that moment. This suggests that affect can incite as well as obstruct our capacities to feel, act and understand. I also suggest that at the organ procurement surgery though I may have been unable to operate in that moment, the encounter precipitated feelings of discomfort and bewilderment, inquiring thoughts, a desire to understand why, which led to an enhancement of my practice and subsequent ideas on training in the days, months and years that followed. Therefore, the question arises as to whether the effects of states of affectation can persist long after the encounter? If so, what is the nature of the relationship between the flows of affect that arise and the precipitating event? Are they inextricably connected?

2.3   What are the qualities associated with affect?

To develop these initial concepts of affect I turn to Melissa Gregg and Gregory Seigworth who provide the best short account of affect that I have come across in recent years:

> Affect arises in the midst of *in-between-ness*: in the capacities to act and be acted upon. Affect is an impingement or extrusion of a momentary or sometimes more sustained state of relation *as well as* the passage (and the duration of passage) of forces or intensities. That is, affect is found in those intensities that pass from body to body (human, nonhuman, part-body, and otherwise), in those resonances that circulate about, between, and sometimes stick to bodies and worlds, *and* in the very passages or variations between those intensities and resonances themselves. Affect, at its most anthropomorphic, is the name we give to those forces – visceral forces beneath, alongside, or generally *other than* conscious knowing, vital forces existing beyond emotion – that can serve to drive us toward movement, toward thought and extension, that can likewise suspend us (as if in neutral) across a barely registering accretion of force-relations, or that can leave us overwhelmed by the world's apparent intractability. Indeed, affect is persistent proof of a body's never less than ongoing immersion in and among the world's obstinacies and rhythms, its refusals as much as its invitations.
>
> (2010, p. 1, original emphasis)

Despite the brevity of this concise description, there are at least five points that I wish to consider. Each is presented as a short summary and then a more in-depth discussion for those readers who choose to delve further.

Affective forces are intensities, non-conscious and prior to emotion

Summary

Gregg and Seigworth emphasize the nature of affect as an 'intensity', referring to how it is a force that drives us to feel: 'affect isn't what I feel, so much as it is what forces me to feel' (Shaviro 2016). As such, affect is a *surge of energy, a rush*, not necessarily conscious, but from which conscious experience may arise and therefore affect functions to inform experiences – impels us to feel, think or act in certain ways. It arises prior to consciousness, with no connection to our individual autobiographies or past experiences and for that reason is 'pre-personal'. Emotion on the other hand, as discussed earlier, is a display of feeling that emanates from an individual's prior and personal experiences (biographical) (Shrouse 2005).

I share here how I initially conceptualised affect through the infant days of my first-born son, Mahen. This approach is informed by the writings of Daniel Stern (1985), whose research on the relationship between mother and infant led to his theory of 'affective attunement' (Stern 1985; Stern et al. 1987).

Mahen's arrival in this world taught me to *see* things in a manner that I had not done since my days as a small child, most likely. Many parents will experience, as I did, how those first days at home with a newborn are fascinating. I watched him squirm, cry or wrinkle his tiny face in displeasure, see the curl of his lips hint at a smile when fat and contented upon being fed. He was awash with physical expressions of what he experienced at any moment in time, a necessary survival strategy given the lack of vocabulary or verbal skill to convey his needs. By studying this display of *affect*, I learnt about my child and his initial experiences of the world. I developed an acute sensitivity to his demeanour and how he would communicate his needs even before they became conscious thoughts. Mahen had no vocabulary, autobiography or previous experiences to drawn on to describe the sensations that coursed through his body. However, these *felt experiences* of the world were pure affect.

Further discussion

Although affect is described as an 'intensity', which lies beyond our own conscious reach, this does not imply that affect cannot be 'reached' or 'touched' and thereby manipulated and taken advantage of by other factors in the contexts of our lives. Indeed, it is the capacity of affect to be manipulated, or to be touched by way of manipulating our consciously known choices of thought and action, that is one of the key interests in this book. Affect is responsible for making us feel feelings, where 'feelings' refer to the experience of sensations checked against previous such encounters. Brian Massumi, a Canadian philosopher and writer, who has written extensively on the subject of affect, describes affect, in contrast to emotion, as a 'pre-personal intensity' (Deleuze and Guattari 1987, p. xvi).

In an earlier statement, Gregg and Seigworth propose that affect is 'vital forces existing beyond emotion – that can serve to drive us toward movement, toward thought and extension, that can likewise suspend us (as if in neutral) across a barely registering accretion of force-relations, or that can leave us overwhelmed by the world's apparent intractability'. These emerging new *intensities* of experience ('vital forces') intimately *connect* the learner to the encounter with practice, so that affect can be contemplated both in terms as something that drives us towards a way of being but at the same time constitute our experience of that 'something'. To return to the example of the organ procurement narrative, the affective forces that arise from my encounter with a deceased patient, precipitates what I described earlier as the *speechlessness of experience* – a mute and paralysed state – but this physical expression of my affective state is also my experience of this bewildering event of practice.

Before concluding this section, I want to return to Daniel Stern's theory of affective attunement briefly, as it has useful pedagogic implications. Stern observed that a mother matches some aspect of emotion seen in her infant child in specific 'external ways', for example touching, smiling and cuddling. He asserted that what is reflected by the mother is the infant's *inner state of emotion* not the infant's physical response. These qualities cannot be easily captured by the 'static' vocabulary used to describe categories of emotion such as 'sadness' or 'joy'. The mother's actions create a preverbal understanding of affective states, signifying a form of implicit relational knowing (Stern 1985, p. 57). Therefore, affective attunement can reinforce and affirm an unconscious inner state, which may reflect a true sense of self at a given moment. Developing pedagogic strategies that are built around an awareness or implementation of these ideas can support efforts to draw alongside the learner experience.

The dual nature of affect: to affect and in turn be affected

Summary

Gregg and Seigworth emphasise the 'in-between-ness' of affect, which essentially refers to its dual ability to impel thoughts and actions that may be consciously undertaken ('to act/to affect') *as well as* condition and prepare us for what is to come in ways that are not consciously understood ('to be acted on/to be affected by'). This resonates with Benedict de Spinoza's construction of affect as a couplet (1996). In essence, he states that when one entity (human or non-human) encounters another entity in ways that expand its capacity to act, this constitutes a heightened capacity *to affect* and in turn *be affected*.

An example of this state of affectations is the story of my first organ retrieval surgery in Chapter 1. I affect the encounter with the deceased patient through my position as a surgeon – I contemplate the human life in front of me through medical parameters (blood pressure, heart rate, does she have any medical conditions that may affect the quality of her organs?) and (necessarily) medicalise her existence, an inevitable consequence of the operative environment. However, in return I am affected by the patient and the event of organ retrieval surgery. My speechless and paralysed state reflects this initial affective engagement with the encounter and then in the days, weeks and months that follow, this affectation expands my abilities to understand and conceive my practice as a transplant surgeon leading to me developing new ways to contemplate how to teach in surgical environments.

Further discussion

As affect is an expression of how a particular event impacts an individual, it represents how that individual initially, though unconsciously, attempts to structure the unknown experience because it represents that individual's attempts to grasp the unfamiliar substance of the encounter and the chaos of the experience. In this way affect represents an inherent *form* to an encounter.

At present, and as is argued in this book, external schemes are brought to bear on experiences of learning and practice in an effort to organise and provide structure to the messiness of the encounter – this is the notion of hylomorphism, introduced in the previous chapter. However, what I argue here is that the emerging affective intensities in and of themselves structure the encounter, reflecting how that event of practice becomes significant for that particular individual – how *I first come to know the event*, or put another way, how the encounter comes to *matter to me*: to my being, my person and ultimately my practice.

Affective experiences can leave us unable to act or extraordinarily capable

Summary

At any point human beings are subject to the internal wranglings that can equally prompt action as well as obstruct it. Brian Massumi describes this situation as a 'diminished or augmented state of capacitation' (Massumi 2008, p. 2). 'Augmented state' refers to *what I can do which is at the limits of my capacities in a given moment*, whereas a diminished state relates to an inability or incapacity to cope, think or act, a disengagement when confronted by something unfamiliar or unknown.

Further discussion

Augmented and diminished states are present in the example of hearing the difficulties encountered with Mr. Martino's treatment from Mary Ellen, a staff member. I can make the decision to talk to Mr. Martino and risk his potential wrath and my feelings of discomfort and unease ('augmented' state) or walk out of the room as soon as I sense his disengaged stance and leave other staff members to manage his care ('diminished' state). Suffice to say that there are times when walking away from a potentially unhelpful and tense encounter is the better option to avoid unnecessary conflict, but what I emphasize here is how an 'augmented state' relates to the efforts made to advance our capacities to cope when confronted by complex events of practice. The transition to a state of enhanced abilities or capacities to see, think and act is not necessarily confined by time, meaning that if I had chosen to walk away on this particular occasion, but reflected and returned at some other time to engage with the difficult patient interaction, this would still constitute a move towards an 'augmented state'.

It is easy to objectify the two options I choose between ('engaging with patient' and 'not engaging with patient') by assuming that I rationalise the situation and make a judgement between them. However, these options represent my 'drives' (Deleuze and Guattari 1983, adopt Nietzsche's original term, cited in *Daybreak* 1881) or what Leibniz calls 'motives' and 'inclinations'. They represent what my innate tendencies, inclinations or orientations are in this situation. My inclinations are motifs that run through my being and which can be modulated by the constituent parts of the encounter, which include the sight of an abundance of delicious food, the warm aroma of dessert to my hungry palate, the draw of Mr. Martino's bed on my fatigued body, the visual image of the patient's lean and jaundiced frame, the light and shade in the room, the phone in my pocket, the sound of Mrs. Martino's sobs, the ticking clock, the knowledge that irate staff are waiting in theatre, Mr. Martino refusing to acknowledge me, my growing sense of desperation (and other things that are not consciously perceptible to me). While I register these events, I am not conscious of the intensities they precipitate. However, the affective relations that form and develop in the encounter become visible through the consequent ways in which I think, emote and behave.

How I eventually behave is a result of the tussle I experience between the feelings that are agitating and to some degree tormenting me. Massumi (2008) suggests that at any one moment as individuals we have no fixed identity ('pre-constituted'), instead we are 'pre-populated' by feelings, memories, inclinations, drives. We emerge as subjects through the act of experiencing, where affect is a dimension of this event. Although affect arises as a consequence of a specific experience, once formed it is autonomous and independent of the very thing that precipitated it in the first place – affect is an unstructured force, independent of any content.

Affective forces brace us for what is to come

Summary

In moments of unforeseen and unpredictable events of clinical practice, processes of affecting and being affected can create tiny interruptions – 'microshocks' (McKim 2008, p. 4) – to the ways in which our lives were proceeding up until that moment. Our bodies act like *resonating chambers* for the emerging affects that flow from an encounter – and which constitute the context of the encounter – bringing about a change or difference to our lives. This 'in-bracing' (Massumi 2008) relates to the attempts the body makes to respond to a given circumstance, preparing for what may come next. It is not the same as an instinct or gut feeling, which are consciously experienced sensations, though these phenomena may be the *effects of* affective in-bracing.

Microshocks are not necessarily detected or identified when they are generated by an encounter. However, what is noticeable or perceptible are their effects which can manifest in many ways, such as determined speech or action on the one hand and on the other an incapacity to exert a consciously experienced response (an example is my mute and paralysed state at the organ retrieval surgery).

Further discussion

An illustration of this idea relates to how I am affected by Mr. Martino's disengagement and lack of eye contact with the occupants of the room. The resultant microshocks cause me to alter my trajectory on a busy operating day – I switch off my phone, and then reflect on how the theatre team will attempt to call me for the next surgery. I brace myself for a potentially difficult interaction with Mr. Martino, at this point although I have a sense of unease, I cannot foresee how this encounter will actually unravel. In these moments of encounter, as Jeff Martino and I both in-brace (he too is being affected – on this occasion by me in my position as his doctor and carer) all there is in that instant is the 'affective hit'.

> You own the feeling as your own, and recognise it as a content in your life, an episode in your personal history. But in the instance of the affective hit, there is no content yet. All there is is the affective quality, coinciding with the feeling of the interruption . . . it takes over life, fills the world, for an immeasurable instant of shock.
>
> (Mckim 2008, p. 5)

The multitude of responses (emotions, thoughts, actions), reactions (anger, fury, pity) and outcomes (strategies to feed and nourish the patient, perhaps a pause in the chemical treatments to provide Mr. Martino a break from the medicalisation of his life) that will be instigated through these affective encounters are yet to be determined in that moment of the 'affective hit'. During these moments our bodies enfold the context of an encounter, bracing ourselves for the unknown.

Affects are independent and autonomous

Summary

As affects form and develop within a particular encounter, they also become *independent of the encounter* which originally brought them into existence (Deleuze and Guattari 1994, p. 164). An example from the organ procurement story in the introductory chapter is how in the days and months that follow the encounter with the deceased donor, the affects precipitated by the specific conditions of that event are still present, even though the encounter itself has passed.

These affective intensities emerged from my non-conscious attempts to grasp the encounter and make sense of it. They bring into being emotions that comprise bewilderment, anxiety, grief, guilt and sadness (regarding the patient's tragic demise), they influence my thoughts and behaviours about the realities of transplant surgery and the challenges and responsibilities of responding as a professional against my feelings and concerns as a fellow human being.

Thus, affective states can occupy contradictory positions, existing both as remnants of the initial encounter with the patient and at the same time exerting an independence from the precipitating event.

What is the significance of these persisting affective components? Why do they matter? Affective intensities and resonances condition beliefs, thoughts and behaviours, influencing the ways in which practice is conceived and carried out, long after the initiating event has passed.

Further discussion

Brian Massumi (2002, 2015) and others (Berelson and Murphie 2010) have warned that ignoring the effect of affective intensities is dangerous, because it conceals the harm that manipulating affective lives can engender. Massumi in his book *Ontopower: war, powers and the state of perception* (2015) explores this quality of affect further using the events and discourses around '9/11': the collapse of the twin towers in New York following systematic terrorist attacks.

> What was striking in the aftermath of 9–11 was the radicality of the shift to that dimension of affective operation, expressed in the compulsive fascination with the endlessly repeated images of the disaster. The shift didn't come through words, but in a being agape, being at a loss for words – it came of that affective cut in the very possibility of discourse.[1]

He argues that the repeated images of the towers being attacked and subsequently collapsing were played relentlessly on news and other media for days and months after the event. People were seen to be watching these images upright and agape. There was no tolerance for a discussion around what factors may have been implicated in the possible motivations underlying that attack. Instead, the affective states were cultivated around discussions of horror and shock. It created an 'affective cut' in political discourse, laying the groundwork for a foreign policy of pre-emptive attack. He concludes from his analysis that politics is distinguished by how it acts to capture and manipulate affective states. He theorises that in the days and months after the terrorist attack, the Bush administration forged enduring and powerful links with the affective states that erupted, leading to a political rhetoric around notions of security.

It could be argued that the images are powerful because of the emotions they galvanise. However, Massumi asserts that emotions would not be stirred if the images did not first have the capacity to generate affective states:

> Affect is autonomous to the degree to which it escapes confinement in the particular body whose vitality, or potential for interaction, it is. Formed, qualified, situated perceptions and cognitions fulfilling functions of actual connections or blockage are the capture and closure of affect. Emotion is the most intense (most contracted) expression of that *capture* – and of the fact that something has always and again escaped.
>
> (Massumi 2002, p. 35)

The cultural critic Eric Shrouse (2005) states that:

> The importance of affect rests upon the fact that in many cases the message consciously received may be of less import to the receiver of that message than his or her non-conscious affective resonances with the source of the message.

Shrouse emphasises the power of affect as insidious and more potent than the effects of an explicit message which is processed consciously. He concludes by stating that the power of many forms of media lie, 'not so much in their ideological effects, but in their ability to create affective resonances independent of content or meaning'. A comprehensive understanding of the power of affect can also create the potential for ethical creativity and transformation, or equally ethical manipulation and coercion.

2.4   Can affects be experienced differently?

The short answer to this question is 'yes'. To return to the story of Mr. Martino, four individuals inhabit the same affective environment (a cocktail of bodily decay, human despair and the rich aroma of freshly cooked food) in which the affects generated during the encounter were *felt differently* and responded to in different ways. Martino is both withdrawn and furious, his wife and son are exasperated and desperate, whilst I am guilty and fatigued.

Massumi explains that what happens in an event is distributed across all those bodies: 'each body will carry a different set of tendencies and capacities, there is no guarantee that they will act in union even if they are cued in concert' (2002, p. 6). He goes on to conclude that 'we're all in on the event together, but we're in it together differently' (Manning et al. 2011, np).

I suggest that healthcare workers are continually braced for events. However, how these in-bracings are then experienced and the responses they create vary from individual to individual. Massumi cites the outcome as in part due to the different set of tendencies, prior experiences, habits and beliefs we 'bring with us' to the encounter. In short, how we collectively inbrace the affects may be attuned, but our responses to the affective experiencing is different.

The question then arises as to how it may be possible to capture the intensity of the in-bracing, so that there can be more solidarity and affective coordination between the group. What I am querying is how it is possible in clinical learning environments to affectively attune with the learner or draw alongside the trainee's experience. Such an affective correlation between trainee and trainer may have a few important implications for learning. First, from a trainer's perspective it may provide an improved ability to recognise and understand what the learner is experiencing. The learner's experience of a training encounter may not be reflected in the established teaching practices. Second, as discussed earlier, affective attunement may enhance pedagogic strategies aimed at supporting learners engaged in contingent and complex practice. Third, it may also facilitate a learner's exploration of the event to identify new ways of thinking and acting that may emerge from the experience of clinical practice.

2.5   Affective experiences: what are the implications for developing an ethics of practice?

At the beginning of this chapter I raised a point regarding how my actions and conduct in the encounter with Mr. Martino may be viewed as unprofessional or inappropriate. Other clinicians confronted with the same encounter may have responded differently. For example, another surgeon may attribute Mr. Martino's attitude and behaviour to depression and proceed to find an appropriate therapy (psychiatric referral, prescription of anti-psychotics etc.). Others may have walked out of the room wishing to avoid a difficult conversation or decided to 'cheer him up' with humour or promises of improved health or confronted him angrily about his 'non-compliance' or gone away to read up on new cures for organ rejection and so on. What I draw attention to is how emotions and actions can emerge from unexpected encounters which are a product of how the affective resonance of an experience is perceived and felt.

With such potential variation in how the effects of affect can manifest, what does this mean for developing and promoting professional codes of conduct or an ethics of practice?

> Perhaps most importantly, we must recognise that ethics requires us to risk ourselves at moments of unknowingness, when what forms us diverges from what lies before us, when our willingness to become undone in relation to others constitutes our chance of becoming human. To become undone by another is a primary necessity, an anguish to be sure, but also a chance – to be addressed, claimed, bound to what is not me, but also to be moved, to be prompted to act, to address myself elsewhere, and so to vacate the self-sufficient 'I' as a kind of possession. If we speak and try to give an account from this place, we will not be irresponsible, or, if we are, we will surely be forgiven.
>
> (Butler 2005, p. 136)

In this quotation by Judith Butler, ethics is imagined as more than a code of behaviour or conduct; it is an ethics relative to how one responds and emerges in the 'thisness' of the clinical encounter with all its inherent uncertainty. '*Moments of unknowingness*' relate to the occasions where one struggles to work out how to proceed given the absence of appropriate guidance or reference to prior knowledge or experience. It is the task of engaging with the unfamiliar. Ethical codes are necessary in formulating guidelines, but often, due to unexpected events of practice, they become inadequate. In these situations, it may be necessary to 'risk ourselves', that is, to embrace the uncertainty of the encounter with a view to responding in ways that exceed what is known. Such a response, I argue, is intimately connected to the affective conditions of the experience. These arguments are further developed in the next chapters.

Note

1 Taken from 'Q&A with Brian Massumi': https://dukeupress.wordpress.com/2015/08/19/qa-with-brian-massumi/ accessed on 21 August 2018.

References

Artino, R. A., and Naismith, L. M. (2015). " 'But how do you really feel?' Measuring Emotions in Medical Education Research." *Medical Education*, 49: 138–146.

Berelson, L., and Murphie, A. (2010). "An Ethics of Everyday Infinities and Powers: Felix Guattari on Affect and the Refrain." In Seigworth, G. J., and Gregg, M. (Eds.), *The Affect Theory Reader*. Durham, NC: Duke University Press.

Blanchette, I., and Richards, A. (2010). "The Influence of Affect on Higher Level Cognition: A Review of Research on Interpretation, Judgement, Decision Making and Reasoning." *Cognition and Emotion*, 24 (4): 561–595.

Breuer, J., and Freud, S. (2001 (1893)). "On the Psychical Mechanism of Hysterical Phenomena (J. Strachey, Trans.)." In Strachey, J., and Freud, A. (Eds.), *The Standard Edition of the Complete Psychological Works of Sigmund Freud, Volume II* (pp. 1–17). London: Vintage Books.

Butler, J. (2005). *Giving an Account of Oneself*. Fordham University Press.

Coulter, A., and Collins, A. (2011). "Making Shared Decision-Making a Reality: No Decision About Me, Without Me." *London: The King's Fund*, 1–40.

Damasio, A. (2000). *The Feeling of What Happens: Body, Emotion and the Making of Consciousness*. London: Vintage Books.

Deleuze, G. and Guattari, F. (1977). *Anti-Oedipus*, trans. Hurley, R., Seem, M., and Lane, H. New York: Viking.

Deleuze, G., and Guattari, F. (1983). *On the Line*. New York: Semiotext(e) Inc.

Deleuze, G. and Guattari, F. (1987). *A Thousand Plateaus: Capitalism and Schizophrenia*. University of Minnesota Press.

Deleuze, G., and Guattari, F. (1994). *What Is Philosophy?* trans. Tomlinson, H., and Burchell, G. New York: Fordham University Press.

Dornan, T., Pearson, E., Carson, P., Helmich, E., and Bundy, C. (2015). "Emotions and Identity in the Figured World of Becoming a Doctor." *Medical Education*, 49: 174–185.

Ekman, P. (2007). *Emotions Revealed*. New York: St Martin's Griffin.

Epstein, R. M., and Street, R. L. (2011). "The Values and Value of Patient-Centred Care." *Annals of Family Medicine*, 9: 100–103.

Farquhar, J., Kamei, R., and Vidyarthi, A. (2018). "Strategies for Enhancing Medical Student Resilience: Student and Faculty Member Perspectives." *International Journal of Medical Education*, 9: 1–6.

Harding, E., Wait, S., and Scruton, J. (2015). "The State of Play in Person-Centred Care: Pragmatic Review of How Person-Centred Care Is Defined, Applied and Measured, Featuring Selected Key Contributors and Case Studies Across the Field." *The Health Foundation*, 1–140.

Hawkes, N. (2015). "Seeing Things from the Patients' View: What Will It Take?" *The British Medical Journal*, 3350: g7757.

Howe, A., Smajdor, A., and Stockl, A. (2012). "Towards an Understanding of Resilience and Its Relevance to Medical Training." *Medical Education*, 46: 349–356.

Immordino-Yang, M. H., and Damasio, A. (2007). "We Feel, Therefore We Learn: The Relevance of Affective and Social Neuroscience to Education." *Mind, Brain Education*, 1 (1): 3–10.

Izard, C. E. (2009). "Emotion Theory and Research: Highlights, Unanswered Questions, and Emerging Issues." *Annual Review of Psychology*, 60: 1–25.

Krathwohl, D. R., Bloom, B. S., and Masia, B. B. (1973). *Taxonomy of Educational Objectives, the Classification of Educational Goals. Handbook II: Affective Domain*. New York: David McKay Co., Inc.

Leibniz, G. W. (2008). *New Essays on Human Understanding*, eds. Remnant, P., and Bennett, J. New York: Cambridge University Press.

Lief, H. I., and Fox, R. C. (1963). "Training for 'detached concern' in Medical Students." In Lieff, H. I., Lieff, V. F., and Lieff, N. R. (Eds.), *The Psychological Basis for Medical Practice*. New York: Harper & Rowe.

MacLeod, A. (2011). "Caring, Competence and Professional Identities in Medical Education." *Advances in Health Sciences Education, Theory and Practice*, 16 (3): 375–394.

Manning, E., Massumi, B., et al. (2011). "Affective attunement in a field of catastrophe". Available on: http://www.peripeti.dk/2012/06/06/affective-attunement-in-a-field-of-cata strophe/ (Accessed: 23 July 2016).

Massumi, B. (2002). *Parables for the virtual*. Durham, NC: Duke University Press..

Massumi, B. (2008). "The Thinking-Feeling of What Happens." *A Semblance of a Conversation*. Retrieved from http://inflexions.org/n1_The-Thinking-Feeling-of-What-Hap pens-by-Brian-Massumi.pdf.

Massumi, B. (2015). *Ontopower: Wars, Power and the State of Perception*. Duke University Press.

McAllister, M., and McKinnon, J. (2009). "The Importance of Teaching and Learning Resilience in the Health Disciplines: A Critical Review of the Literature." *Nurse Education Today*, 29: 371–379.

McConnell, M. M., and Eva, K. W. (2012). "The Role of Emotion in the Learning and Transfer of Clinical Skills and Knowledge." *Academic Medicine*, 87 (10): 1–7.

McKim, J. (2008). *Of Microperception and Micropolitics: An Interview with Brian Massumi*, 15 August. Retrieved from www.inflexions.org/n3_Of-Microperception-and-Mic ropolitics-An-Interview-with-Brian-Massumi.pdf.

McNaughton, N. (2013). "Discourse(s) of Emotion Within Medical Education: The Ever-Present Absence." *Medical Education*, 47: 71–79.

Nietzsche, F. (1982). *Daybreak: Thoughts on the Prejudices of Morality*, trans. Hollingdale, R. J. Cambridge: Cambridge University Press.

Schutz, P. A., and Pekrun, R. (2007). "Introduction to Emotion in Education." In Schutz, P. A., and Pekrun, R. (Eds.), *Emotion in Education: A Volume in Educational Psychology* (pp. 3–10). Cambridge, MA: Academic Press, Elsevier Inc.

Seigworth and M. Gregg (Eds), *The Affect Theory Reader*. Durham NC: Duke University Press.

Shapiro, J. (2011). "Perspective: Does Medical Education Promote Professional Alexithymia? A Call for Attending to the Emotions of Patients and Self in Medical Training." *Academic Medicine*, 86: 326–332.

Shaviro, S. (2016). Affect/Emotion. Available at: http://www.shaviro.com/Blog/?p=1366 (Accessed 12 June 2016).

Shrouse, E. (2005). *Feeling, Emotion, Affect*. Retrieved from http:culture.org.au/0512/03-shouse.php (Accessed 24 July 2016).

Spinoza, B. (1996). Ethics. London: Penguin.

Stern, D. N. (1985). *The Interpersonal World of the Infant*. New York: Basic Books.

Stern, D. N., Hofer, L., et al. (1987). "Affective Attunement: Division of Emotional States Between Mother and Child by Cross-Modal Exchange." *Annales Medico-Psychologiques* (Paris), 145 (3): 205–224.

Stewart, K. (2007). *Ordinary Affects*. Durham, NC: Duke University Press.

3 Exploring Experiences of Learning and Practice

pedagogies of encounter

> Conceptual frameworks are like lighthouses and lenses. . . . Whereas the lighthouse illuminates certain parts of the ocean at any given time, other parts are left in the dark. Each framework highlights or emphasises different aspects of a problem or research question. . . . Any one conceptual framework presents only a partial view of reality. By contrast, conceptual frameworks are also like magnifying glasses; each individual framework magnifies certain elements of the problem.
>
> (Bordage 2009, p. 313)

3.1 Chapter objectives: developing a theory of knowing from the inside

This chapter is concerned with promoting and cultivating interconnections between theory and actual practice. In it I develop a conceptual framework to theorise practice – each framework examines the matter from a particular theoretical perspective and therefore provides what Georges Bordage describes as a 'partial view of reality'. The objective of conceptual frameworks is to deepen awareness and understanding through theoretical scrutiny. Whilst bringing a particular aspect of practice into focus, such a theoretical lens can also paradoxically 'open up' *actual* events of clinical practice (an exploration of practice without prejudgements) to illuminate the multiple realities that can emerge from these learning encounters. In this way, theory is not used to structure practice, replicating the hylomorphism that I have spent the last two chapters cautioning against! Instead, the uncertain character of practice informs the theoretical approach I take, so that learning encounters can be explored from the perspective of how they are initially experienced.

What I suggest and develop in this chapter is a pedagogy that attempts to work with the notion of a kind of *knowing on the inside* as it emerges from within events of practice. Such an approach *does not* presuppose a particular subject of knowledge, one that is grounded in an epistemology created from past experiences. Whereas, in the process of knowing on the inside, or *knowing which is immanent to events*, knowing and the subject are not prior, established entities – they do not pre-date the encounter with a particular event of learning or practice – instead they emerge through the flux of experiencing that constitutes this encounter.

These ideas are best contemplated through the example of a waterfall, used by Dennis Atkinson (2018) to illustrate the power of affect in art practice. He describes the unique dual experiences of *standing in* a waterfall and the states of affect that emerge from within compared to the experience of *standing outside* on the banks of a river and watching the waterfall, observing it (ibid., p. 122). Caught in the strong rushes of water standing within the waterfall, the force of the flows of water can trigger powerful affective states: the crashing flows of water may leave one utterly terrified or supremely exhilarated. This lies in stark contrast to the affect precipitated by the act of watching the tumbling torrents of water from the riverbanks. One may still feel a sense of thrill or fear but the *local intensity of the experience* is different to the flows of experience that come about as an observer. Standing within the waterfall represents the *immanent nature of experience*, capturing the flows of affect and emotion.

3.2　What is pedagogy of encounter?

The waterfall analogy illustrates how we experience something in the moment in contrast to how we experience it later when recalling, recollecting and reflecting on something. The immanence of being inside an encounter is not the same as the immanence of observation (Atkinson 2018, p. 122). The latter also applies to how teachers observe or assess a trainee – they cannot know how the trainee experiences or feels events of practice, they can only draw conclusions from what is visible or demonstrable.

Pedagogy of encounter (POE) attempts to capture the intensity of the learner/ practitioner experience as it emerges from the substance of the event itself. This pedagogic approach introduces different yet complementary ways of considering how unanticipated encounters of clinical practice can inform the knowledge or knowing that arises from an event. The objective is to discover what can be inferred about the nature of pedagogic relations and opportunities embedded within real experiences of clinical training.

POE follows the seminal research that has come before on relevant theories of learning – tacit knowing (Polanyi 1958, 2009), communities of practice (Lave and Wenger 1991), experiential learning (Kolb 1984) and reflection-in-action (Schon 1983), to name a few – and attempts to go beyond expressed communication and observable behaviours, which are visible and demonstrable aspects of learning in clinical settings. It aims to theorise the *unseen and unspoken elements* of actual events of practice from which arise affective forces that are difficult to anticipate and predict (described in the first chapter as the 'speechlessness of experience').

POE builds on the critical discussions of affect in the last chapter and attempts to loosen the ideological framings that currently structure medical education and practice, for example competency-based medical education and the dominant discourses that frame thinking and learning as primarily cognitive and rational processes. What I hope to introduce in these pages is a set of theoretical tools that can work alongside existing transcendent knowledge and practice, acknowledging their critical importance whilst functioning as a complementary pedagogy to interrogate the individual nature of lived encounters of practice.

This mode of enquiry resonates with the emerging literature on the importance of sociomaterial methodologies in medicine (Fenwick 2014; Dall Jensen et al. 2018) which treat the learner and the learning environment as inseparable, *a duality*, intimately connected, resisting attempts to be constructed as distinct entities (Kemmis et al. 2014; Buch and Andersen 2015). Dall Jensen et al. (2018) conclude that 'the education of surgeons needs to take the *sayings, doings and relatings* that constitute a surgical practice into account when preparing students to perform in their future workplace' (p.861, my emphasis). Adopting a philosophical lens to explore the affective nature of *experience* and *experiencing* requires an approach that is sufficiently nuanced to accommodate and account for the human lives within which unpredictable clinical events occur. Such an approach permits an exploration of the multiple realities embedded in encounters of practice, whilst deepening the understanding of relations of the self and of practice, the construction of values that mediate and shape what is understood and an appreciation of the knowledge created through *intra-actions* (Barad 2007) between the knower and known. Simply put, 'intra-actions' refer to the complex layers of relations and connections that form and develop between the living subject (the knower – the learner/practitioner) and non-living subject (the known).

A philosophical framework to problematise experiences of clinical training permit an approach that is more 'open' and not subject to fixed criteria (Shaviro 2012; Atkinson 2016). Put another way, I advocate a research framework that avoids examining any particular clinical experience from pre-established notions and transcendent categories. It has the potential to consider dimensions of practice that are not immediately self-evident and may otherwise remain *invisible* or even be perceived as *'harmful'* by the dominant biomedical discourses in medicine. My intention is twofold: to support and facilitate a learner to understand her modes of learning and to help educators orient and conceive their teaching practices.

3.3   Entangled subjectivities

In the following account, Radha, a consultant surgeon based at a teaching hospital outside of London, describes an encounter with a seriously ill patient during her on-call. What is most striking in her narrative is how the various elements that constitute her on-call encounter with the surgical patient – the emotional pull of her family commitments, the personal impact of the patient's harrowing story of medical trauma and her attempts to provide a surgical solution, her run-in with a colleague, her personal thoughts and feelings about the multiple roles she inhabits during this encounter, her strategies for coping with the harsh realities of her practice and life as a private individual – construct her *sense of self* and professional identity. That is, her emerging subjectivities in practice. The term 'subjectivity' refers to a sense of self or a concept of self-identity. Chapter 6 explores in more depth the theme of subjectivities in clinical practice and training.

I use Radha's narrative to highlight the five aspects of learning encounters that concern the theoretical discussion of this chapter.

First, the prevailing conception of thinking and doing in medical education as primarily cognitive processes of reasoning and rationality. This paradigm of learning excludes other, less demonstrable processes of *making sense* which may signify how learning encounters or events of practice come to assume importance or become meaningful for an individual.

Second, the treatment of uncertainty in medical education and clinical research which emphasises the development of strategies to minimize the contingency of medical encounters whilst the modes of *being* and *becoming* that can emerge from unanticipated events are neither prioritised nor explored.

Third, the state of affectations precipitated by the immanence of clinical events – how one can affect and in turn be affected by the thisness of practice.

Fourth, the entangled relations that arise from the ways in which one is *obligated* in practice. This refers to the various relations that form and develop within the encounter as an individual grapples with the event of practice and how it matters to her in an attempt to respond to the event.

Finally, the ways of responding to the haecceities of practice – the thoughts, speech and actions that constitute professional practice and which cultivate a personal ethics of practice, where ethics is conceived beyond a moral code.

3.4   Radha's story

To think that we are unemotional creatures is not true. Our emotion and mental being affects our operating. You know, on days when I know I'm going to be operating, I don't fight with the children that morning, no arguments, just a chilled breakfast. I get into my Zen, because that operating checklist that we go through before starting any procedure, asks right at the end, "is everyone well in the team? Is there anything bothering the team that's going to affect the surgical operations?" That's an important one. And I would put my hand up and declare that I have been up all night on-call, or I've got to make sure I'm out of here by 6 because I've got my child's whatever-it-is-event this evening and I can't miss it. I think that emotional state is important, you know. So, I make sure that I'm unburdened before I start any kind of surgery.

But there are times when you're operating and all this uncertainty arises, you know like when you're called in to emergencies or another surgeon's operating theatre because they need help, you know they've damaged something or found something unexpected and they need you to help to fix it, sort it out.

I remember going to see a female patient in ITU. She had had a horrendous, horrible, horrible experience and ended up losing her baby and her womb, and she had bled so much. I wasn't present at her original surgery but even just hearing about it was in itself so traumatic. I got told about this woman at 7.45 in the morning to say she was being taken to theatre at any moment. But that morning was my daughter's school assembly, and I was all set to go to it for ten minutes, just ten little minutes. But then I got this call and ran out of the house, sort of half promising her I'd be there, but knowing in my heart that it was going to be impossible. So, I rang my husband from the car and told him to video it or whatever, and my daughter was in tears and refused to speak to me. But it was bothering me that I wasn't going to be there. Then to top it all off, as I walk into the hospital the medical director has a go at me because I haven't rolled up my sleeves, you know, I'm not 'bare below the elbows' and therefore I'm an infection risk!

So, when I started that operation I wanted all of these irritations, disappointments, frustrations out of my head . . . so I basically told the team of doctors who were with me, and for me just telling them about how I felt was enough to get it out of my head. I can't be there, I just can't. I'm on-call and this is my duty, I have to be here for the patient. For me, telling someone else was enough to transfer the guilt if you like and get on with the task at hand. I needed to focus because this patient had suffered a terrible injury, a significant one.

Operating that day, the surgery was very difficult, there were two other surgeons in the room . . . and you realise that you've tried all the manoeuvres that you know about, but NOTHING has worked! Then what do you do? You call for help. . . . You realise at that point that you have to stop. You have to close up, it might be absolutely fine and if you need to go back in, then you need to go back in. If you need to do more investigations, then you need to do more investigations. But that thing of learning to stop, which you do learn in very small ways . . . It's then having to sit it out for the next three days and watch her, all the parameters (urine output, haemoglobin, creatinine) . . .

Do I think about what she's going through? Of course . . . On the drive into work that day and the drive home and days after that, when I see her later in clinic, I can't help but think that she has been through a lot and how can anyone understand what she has been through?! I don't think about it too much in a way, especially when you're dealing with the surgical problem. You have to dissociate it, that emotional bit of it. And dealing with the emotions is the really important bit, because otherwise I think it would overwhelm me. Just hearing about the story starts to make you upset . . . you know . . . as a fellow human being.

Thinking and doing as cognitive processes

Pedagogic attempts to reform and improve medical education and clinical training start from the premise that clinical learning and understanding are primarily rational processes. That is, experiences of clinical practice are principally examined by assessing how well a practitioner can recall, reason and analyse information, demonstrate practical skills and apply logical processes that culminate in effective decision making. These are performative parameters of practice; demonstrable, observable and indicative of cognitive forms of thinking. But what about the non-visible and intangible aspects of pre-cognitive thinking that emanate from clinical encounters? The *'speechlessness of experience'* (see Chapter 1), is an expression of these forms of thinking within encounters signifying how a subject initially grasps an unexpected event of practice, attempting to make sense of it. These immediate experiences can influence and shape an individual's approach to clinical practice beyond the established traditions of knowing and doing.

The impact of uncertainty

Radha's narrative illustrates the uncertain nature of all medical practice. It is impossible to adequately control and fully anticipate how any clinical interaction in the realm of doctor-patient relations may unfold (Greenhalgh 2013, 2014). As discussed in the previous chapter, investigating the impact of *emotions* on decision making and learning in medical environments (McConnell and Eva 2012; McNaughton 2013; Gillespie et al. 2018) is a slowly growing field. However, the research on 'uncertainty' remains predominantly conceived through a biomedical discourse of clinical reasoning (Logan and Scott 1996; West and West 2002; Yuill et al. 2010; Guenter et al. 2011). In this conception of practice, uncertainty can be reduced or eliminated through an application of evidence-based medicine (EBM) or by the standardisation of healthcare processes to create predictability and objective knowledge (Sacket et al. 1996; Timmermans and Berg 2003). Examples include the institution of protocols and pathways in emergency medicine, such as the algorithm outlining the steps of care for the management of the unconscious patient. Therefore, the literature on uncertainty is predisposed to investigating ways to remove the chaos created by uncertain medical events in a concerted effort to establish control over the event itself and therefore the outcome. This has obvious benefits for patient safety and welfare as well as creating conditions that foster and cultivate good team working amongst clinical staff and effective practice.

However, what concerns me in this chapter is *how* the clinician is *affected* by this uncertainty. Radha describes in detail the uncertainty associated with emergency surgery – not knowing how an operation may unfold despite the best application of knowledge, skills and prior experience. What modes of becoming can arise through an affective engagement with the unexpected nature of practice? How can we unpack and theorise the affective impact of contingency in practice to develop appropriate pedagogical strategies even though, paradoxically, we cannot predict when uncertainty will arise? These questions illustrate how theory is interrogated in this chapter.

To be affected and, in turn, affect

Radha's story primarily draws attention to the fluctuating state of affectations that contribute to how a clinician engages in clinical practice at any given moment of time. This relates directly to my initial claims regarding the effects of the affective dimension of clinical encounters. In the first instance, Radha is *affected by* her encounter with the female patient which begins when she is told of the traumas this woman has endured. All the components that constitute this event of practice, such as the first time she meets the patient in the ICU followed later by her struggles in the operating room to arrest the bleeding, initially generate responses that are affective in nature and which compose how she encounters this particular patient in this singular occasion of practice. These first affective impressions, which may not be visible or palpable, impact the way Radha proceeds to see, interpret, know, understand and behave during and beyond this single event of practice.

In turn, Radha *affects* the clinical event through her position as the on-call surgeon: providing medical care for this patient, operating on her, observing and monitoring her in the ICU, making clinical decisions that impact this patient's outcome. At this point it may be useful to think about these processes of affectation through Benedict de Spinoza's (1996) description of knowledge (he actually identified three types). The first type of knowledge, and the one that I am concerned with here, arises from our many encounters of the world, it refers to how we come to know the world through our experiences of it. This resonates with how Radha comes to know the event of practice through the affective composition of the experience. It is knowledge that emerges from the immanence and contingency of the encounter.

Therefore, within clinical events of practice we have no prior understanding of how our bodies can be affected within learning encounters. The experience can precipitate expanded abilities or diminished capacities of thought and action, which in turn influence the beliefs and behaviours that can form and develop. Here, the pedagogic challenge is to develop strategies that can draw alongside a learner's affective experience of an encounter in ways that reflect and support how this event becomes relevant to this particular learner and her modes of learning. It is up to the individual learner/practitioner/teacher to develop appropriate strategies within and following a given experience, but this process should be intrinsic to the singular nature of the particular event of practice.

Entangled relations emerge from actual events of clinical practice

In a given encounter with practice, we are subject to the 'push' and 'pull' of our professional commitments and personal obligations, so much so, it is often difficult to see where one ends and the other begins. Thus, we are continually engaged in a series of encounters of becoming, such that at any given moment in time, what makes us who we are is fluid (changeable). Radha describes the many different roles, responsibilities and relationships that arise, mingle, interrelate, influence, merge and conflict as she encounters a serious event of surgical practice: these are the entangled relations that shape and influence how a doctor thinks and acts in clinical practice. This includes the personal concerns and commitments, professional duties as well as the relationships formed in the working environment with organic (patients, colleagues) and non-organic (operating theatre, wards, medical equipment) aspects of practice. These forces are engaged in a constant exchange, shifting, moving, influencing, working together and separately at any one moment – described earlier as intra-actions (Barad 2007). These connectivities deepen the existing contingency of clinical encounters by adding a further dimension of complexity to events of practice.

Spinoza's second kind of knowledge leads to an understanding of the relations and capacities that constitute our different states of being and is relevant to this notion of entangled relations. Through the intra-actions within this encounter, Radha is constituted in its thisness, in contrast to the transcendent skills and knowledge that traditionally construct what and who a surgeon is. In other words, it is how one emerges from the immediate experience of encountering something (an event, an object, a person) that determines who we are at that moment in time, rather than a reliance on handbooks of practice or clinical guidelines to clearly define roles, responsibilities and expectations of professionals. Reconfiguring clinicians and learners beyond traditional identities to include the dynamic and uncertain relational processes through which they emerge within real examples of practice acknowledges the complexities of actual practice. These relationalities constitute the ways in which we are *obligated* in our encounters with practice. Put simply, the term 'obligations' refers to how the connections that form and develop within an event of practice commit the individual to certain modes of being and acting within that particular encounter and beyond.

An ethics of immanent practice

Radha's narrative emphasises how she contemplates her abilities in relation to the thisness (immanence) of the encounter. She details the various life events that affected her on that day and her awareness of how these factors might impact her ability to discharge her duties as the on-call surgeon. She even discusses the strategies she has developed to help her focus on the task at hand. I suggest that her narrative illustrates an ethics of immanence. That is, in this particular situation, she attempts to expand what she can think and do, thus extending her capacities in clinical practice. Deleuze distinguishes ethics as separate to morality, an established code of conduct which poses the question, 'Is this right or moral'? to judge actions or behaviour. Ethics, according to Deleuze (echoing the work of Spinoza) is not a transcendent framing of conduct but instead relates to the modes of becoming that arise in a particular encounter to ask, '*what can I do or achieve in this situation'?* Put another way, an ethics of immanence moves away from a moral code to embrace a practical stance, asking, 'how can I extend my capacities to think or act more effectively in this situation'? This position does not trivialise the value of moral codes nor is it subject to accusations of relativism (see later in this chapter). Instead I wish to draw attention to how transcendent criteria dominate our thinking and action such that these forms of knowledge may inhibit a learner's true capacity for discovery, action or learning. In pedagogic terms, it is an ethics that takes root in the thisness of situations, prioritising the capacities that emerge from a learner's processes of becoming.

3.5   How is clinical learning currently theorised in medical education?

The research literature on teaching and learning in clinical practice has adapted social theory and educational theory to investigate aspects of medical education.

The field of social theory is interdisciplinary, drawing on disciplines that include philosophy and sociology. The applications of social theory include particular sociological methodologies. One example is the widespread use of reflective practice to structure and organise the curriculum at both the undergraduate and postgraduate levels (GMC 2016; RCS 2014). However, the difficulty arises when reflective practice or other exercises based on sociological methods are applied as external forms of knowledge to categorise the ways of acting and thinking that arise immanently from the clinical encounter. In other words, static formats are used to capture the immanence of clinical learning, which by nature is dynamic and fluid.

Reflective practice and other assessments

This form of contemplative learning is a core component of the system of appraisal and revalidation that determines the licensing of doctors in the UK. Reflective practice was introduced with the purpose of helping practitioners address and learn from the challenges and complexities that arise from unanticipated and unstructured events of practice. However, it is currently applied both in clinical practice and medical education as an exercise in logic and rationality to explain complex medical encounters with the requirement that the learner/practitioner demonstrate learning. In addition, the emphasis, though unintentional, is on the linguistic ability of the practitioner to describe and discuss the reflective event. But, as already discussed in Chapter 1, finding the appropriate vocabulary to describe professional encounters in practice that defy literal description is a challenge, to say the least. In addition, how one encounters clinical experience can involve responses and processes that are not necessarily amenable to rational thought because they arise from the emotional dimension of practice. These issues are common to many practitioners engaged in healthcare who have found themselves in analogous situations, raising similar questions and frustrations with existing supportive practices.

Another example is the case-based discussion (CBD), a staple amongst the growing spectrum of workplace assessment exercises. CBDs are used to assess clinical judgement, decision making and the application of medical knowledge in an encounter of practice (ISC 2016; Phillips and Jones 2015; Phillips et al 2016). This assessment poses four questions based on principles of reflective practice to make the trainee reflect on the clinical encounter. What did I learn from this experience? What did I do well? What do I need to improve or change and how will I achieve it? These questions force the learner into structuring their experience through rational categories of conscious thought, which raises two important points.

First, outside of this prescriptive format for reflection, how else can we access the trainee's abilities to self-evaluate, critique and organise her experience in ways that demonstrate learning, evolving competency and desirable professional traits in practice? Second, how well does this assessment format capture those aspects of the clinical experience which are not easily disclosed or verbalized: the affective responses that arise from the immanence of practice.

In recent decades, the teaching and learning of surgical skills and knowledge has been formalised and strengthened through an application of educational theory. Examples include the notion of 'deliberate practice' or the 'zone of proximal development'. In the former, repetitive practice of specific components of performance are associated with the acquisition of technical expertise (Ericsson et al. 1993). The concept of the 'zone of proximal development' refers to the potential for development that arises when a learner is provided with a teacher's guidance (Vygotsky 1978). An individual's independent ability to problem solve is furthered by such an intervention.

There are many books within medical and healthcare education that closely examine these theories and their applications to modern-day clinical learning and teaching. It is not the objective of this book to reproduce these works or to propose new applications. Instead, I hope in these pages to expand the theoretical discussions that examine emotional dimensions of learning and practice in clinical environments, querying, 'how does an encounter with practice come to matter to a learner/practitioner'? This requires exploration of the conditions that underpin novel ways to contemplate the thinking, doing and being that emerges when engaged in actual experiences of practice.

3.6   Configuring 'experiencing' as 'real learning'

Conceptualising experiencing through a philosophical lens can permit a more in-depth and nuanced interpretation of learning in clinical environs. This may allow for experiences of clinical training to be problematised and explored through an approach that is more 'open' and not subject to fixed criteria (Shaviro 2012; Atkinson 2016). Put another way, I ask that learners and educators avoid examining any particular clinical experience through pre-established notions and transcendent categories.

Returning to Radha's challenging operative experience, it is not uncommon (as in Radha's account) for patients to be taken to surgery only for the original operative plan to be diverted or subverted. In her case, she could not identify the source of bleeding. Persevering with this complicated surgery resonates with Alain Badiou's (2005) writings on event, first discussed briefly in Chapter 1. To recap, Badiou suggests that an 'event' has the power to rupture standard practices and approved knowledge, disclosing heightened abilities to think and act. Radha reports how she stopped operating further on the patient after she exhausted every intervention she knew of. Her knowledge in this area may have been constructed from textbooks, research literature, surgical conferences as well as her prior intra-operative experiences and the information she had gathered from her colleagues' surgical experiences. However, in moments such as these, the specific patient situation demands an approach that marries her existing knowledge with 'facts' that she comes to *know* as a consequence of the 'rupture'. In other words, committing to the *unpredictable twists and turns of* this event of surgery may extend the knowledge that she is already in possession of.

Dennis Atkinson (2011) modifies Badiou's 'event' to involve an encounter which disrupts an individual's current ontological state and modes of representation, her ways of knowing, thinking and acting. Through the event, a 'new subject' emerges, a new ontological and epistemological state is precipitated, which presents new possibilities of being. Badiou suggests that it is in these moments of ontological and epistemological struggle, that we emerge as subjects who acquire newly formed subjectifications. The power of institutions and processes to shape subjectivities is termed 'subjectification'. We pass beyond our routine existences, and act and think in a way that extends what we know and who we become. For Atkinson (2011), *real learning* is 'what learning can be beyond the parameters of reproduction, packaged knowledge, traditional skills and the pragmatic and predictable application of knowledge' (pp. 5–6).

Surgical trainee versus surgeon-in-training

If learners/trainees are viewed as fixed entities (with a predefined identity and skill set), it restricts other possibilities of what they can become or of what it means to be a learner or a teacher. This is a key point, which again highlights the difference between what I propose to call, a *surgical trainee* versus a *surgeon-in-training*. The terminology alludes to different pedagogical approaches: the first is concerned with the induction of established bodies of knowledge whilst the latter relates to the singular experiences and encounters of a surgeon-in-training, through which learning occurs and produces knowledge (also known as 'practical wisdom' or what the Greeks termed 'phronesis'). In a complex situation, when a trainee is unsure of how to proceed, a form of 'knowing' can arise, which assists one's passage through the encounter. In Radha's case, she commits to closely observing and monitoring the patient through medical parameters. From this surveillance of the patient, she hopes to glean vital information about the recovery of the patient, but in addition encountering the uncertain health status of the patient can trigger thoughts or actions about what else she is able to do. Such is the power of experiencing the complexities of *real* practice.

Badiou views this situated form of 'knowing' as inseparable from ethics: it is an *ethics of immanence* (in a similar vein to Spinoza's writings on ethics [1996]). To help me flesh out this concept further, I return to my aforementioned distinction between a 'surgeon-in-training' and a 'surgical trainee.' In contrast, where ethics is viewed in relation to established knowledge, a trainee is 'forced' to make the situation they find themselves in *fit* the framework of formal knowledge. Otherwise, the encounter may be viewed as completely mysterious or irrelevant. For a surgeon-in-training, the ethical code may be strongly influenced by the reality of actual situations he finds himself in. Whereas, a surgical trainee is expected to conduct himself along established moral codes and expressed bodies of knowledge. This notion of ethics has already been discussed in the previous and is further developed in later chapters.

Conceiving experiences in clinical practice which rupture standard practices is to contemplate a pedagogic project 'articulated around the notion of becoming, where real learning is conceived as self-encounter, an event that projects a learner into a new or modified ontological state' (Atkinson 2011, p. 30).

3.7 The nature of 'experience' and 'experiencing': an affect-based theory

The narratives in this book illustrate how learners/surgical trainees and professional surgeons are constituted through the immanence of their experiences in practice. '*Apart from the experiences of subjects there is nothing, nothing, nothing, bare nothingness*', states Alfred North Whitehead (1929, p. 167, my emphasis), for whom the nature of experience is core to his philosophy. In other words, Whitehead asserts that we are constituted only by our experience of things, be they human beings, non-human objects or events. A subject (for example Radha or the patient in the narrative), comes into being *in and through experience*, this is how they emerge into the world. Whitehead denies the ontological privileging of the human subject and instead asserts that the individual emerges as a *product* of the experience (what he terms the 'superject') where the emphasis is on *the encounter with something* and not the human subject as a static entity.

Whitehead reconfigures the individual (subject) in terms of *how she relates* to the environment she finds herself in. This is not the same as the adage, 'we are the products of our environment'. Here, the implication is that the specific environment we live in can influence and shape our beliefs, ideas and actions. However, what Whitehead emphasises is the notion of encounter – how something (a person, an object etc.) is experienced or taken account of in any environment. Through the act of experiencing, a subject while being constituted is also at the same time constantly perishing. By this statement, he intends to emphasise how in any moment of time, no (clinical) event can be re-lived or re-created in the same exact way, because the subject cannot outlive the feelings she experiences at any given moment (Shaviro 2012, p. xii).

Whitehead proposes an *affect* based account of experience: '*the basis of experience is emotional*' (Shaviro 2012, p. 176, my emphasis). His use of the words 'emotion' and 'feeling' communicate notions of 'affect' – every experience of perception is imbued with an 'affective tone', (ibid., 176). A subject first perceives through a bodily response below a threshold of conscious thought: the response is not immediately influenced or organised by cognition or reason. Therefore, *feeling* is a basic condition of experience, both unconscious and significant for how processes of mattering or meaning for an individual can first emerge through affect.

To return to Radha's experience, as the encounter unfolds, she 'becomes' a surgeon through the relations she forms in the workplace and through her actions in the operating theatre. This is not to deny her professional qualifications or training, but to emphasise how *her subjectivity* emerges through the described encounter. For Whitehead, it is through *experiencing* in the world that things come to matter or acquire meaning in that encounter for the subject, emerging as a being in the universe. This notion of *mattering* emanates from the affective dimension before any attempt to explain or translate that experience through language.

The limits of language

Giles Deleuze and Felix Guattari (2004, p. 289) emphasise the difference between the lived nature of encounters and how experience is fixed or tied down in language. Language is situated in a static discourse which cannot fully embrace the dynamic nature of lived experience. Deleuze and Guattari use the example of words, such as 'child' or 'wolf', which create a precise subject with a fixed identity that is intractable: a wolf is an animal, four legged with claws etc. Language also defines a subject in terms of what it can be or become: the wolf is a predator, dangerous, fierce etc. Therefore, these functions of language help facilitate an individual's ability to visualise a subject (like the wolf) and grasp its reality. However, Deleuze and Guattari argue that the universe is constantly in flux, therefore language and any other discourse which interprets the world through static terms is problematic because it fails to acknowledge and capture the dynamism of entities. Instead, they advocate describing entities in terms of *becoming* and as *events*. Thus, we come into existence through our experiences in the world which cannot be captured by predefined identities or the fixed parameters of language.

Thinking as feeling

Whitehead's principle critique of philosophy in general is its overreliance on cognition to explain the nature and basis of experience. For example, he argues that experience itself can create categories of understanding (1929, p.113), as is illustrated by the many narratives in this book – encounters with practice trigger heightened capacities to see and think, from which new behaviours and professional attitudes emerge.

Whitehead positions questions about *what we feel* or *how we feel* at the heart of philosophy over and above a concern with epistemology or ontology (Shaviro 2012, p. 47). To clarify, he understands the notion of 'feeling' as the way in which a *subject accounts for something* or encounters something that makes a difference to her. This difference can arise through language, smell or touch – something that is sensed or, to use Whitehead's term, *prehended*. Prehension relates to how a subject encounters an object, person or event that makes a difference to her.

Prehension therefore is concerned with how the experience matters to the subject and in what forms or states it matters. In the case of Radha, how she *prehends* the patient in the clinic room, connected to monitors and various intravenous therapies, the swollen state of her face and skin, can all be viewed as experiences of prehension. Once in the operating theatre, Radha prehends the open abdomen through the traumatised and injured tissues and viscera, the smells and sights of the surgery and the behaviour of her colleagues in the room. These elements of the encounter and how she grasps the situation in ways that matter to her create the *thisness* of the experience which she may not necessarily be able to translate into language.

Previous similar experiences may influence her prehension of this particular encounter. For example, in my own narrative of the organ procurement (see Chapter 1) it appears that the other members of the team do not share my affective responses to the event. It may be that repeated exposure to the same operation means that their prehension of that particular operation is different to mine. However, what I emphasize here is that prehension is about how, in the moment, the thisness of practice can make a difference to this practitioner.

Whilst I have used living subjects (Radha) to explain prehension, it is worth briefly pointing out that Whitehead considers even inanimate objects as subjects that can prehend. Using the narrative, this would include a scalpel, the operating table, the scrub cap or mask worn by theatre personnel, in addition to the unconscious patient and surgeon. The scalpel in the hand of the surgeon, 'perceives' the firm pressure applied by the index finger of the surgeon, preparing to incise the skin. The surgeon in turn feels the weight of the sharp instrument in her hands and notes the precision with which it cuts: 'the whole universe . . . consists of elements disclosed in the experiences of subjects' (ibid., p. 166). This approach is consistent with Whitehead's refusal to privilege the human subject and instead focuses the discussion on how it is the experience of things or events that matter, not the individual 'doing' the experiencing.

To summarise Whitehead's approach, *thinking within experience is in the first instance sensing or feeling something*. He asserts that experience is defined purely by the physical reaction to an event (ibid., p. 229).

An example is my speechlessness and inaction as responses to the organ procurement surgery in Chapter 1. I cannot accurately rationalise or reason, with complete confidence, why I behaved this way. What I do remember is that my reaction was immediate and automatic and, in that moment, not motivated by *conscious thought*. I have reflected back to this event countless times. It is possible to arrive at a rational explanation for my actions (my first procurement, I was shocked and inexperienced) as is encouraged by reflective practice in medical training. However, reflective activity is currently framed around a search for reason and purpose in interactions. Such an approach is premised on the notion that we are primarily rational and thoughtful beings. Whitehead, however, disabuses the notion of thought as akin to cognition. Instead he (and others) propose that thought can arise experientially or from sentience or cognition: thought can be 'simple physical feelings' (Whitehead 1929, p. 236). Massumi (2002) has gone on to coin the phrase 'thinking-feeling' to express these ideas around non-cognitive notions of thought (see later).

Multiple realities emerge from clinical encounters

The theoretical discussion so far has focused on *how* something is experienced in those immediate moments of encounter rather than submitting this experience to external established categories which are pre-identified as constituting experience. As briefly discussed in the last two chapters, the latter is an example of transcendence – judging or contemplating something from established concepts, perspectives or criteria. In surgical training, transcendent frameworks of practice refer to the established curriculum (the Intercollegiate Surgical Curriculum), the assimilated training practices and the approved forms of assessment. These forms of knowledge and skills are essential to orienting learners in a subject so that they are taught the necessary skills and theory to perform complicated tasks. Crucially transcendent frameworks in medicine help ensure a standard of practice, which has important implications for the safety and wellbeing of patients.

The key point regarding a philosophy of immanence, meanwhile, is that it attempts to capture particular ways of knowing as they emerge from *within practice* rather than exclusively predicating practice upon established criteria or frameworks of knowledge. Immanence places emphasis upon an openness to processes of becoming, their intensities, affects, ways of knowing and seeing in their specific milieus of practice. In Radha's case, when she walked into the hospital to deal with the emergency surgery, she could not have fully known with certainty what would unfurl: she would be chastised by the medical director, disappoint her daughter by not going to the school assembly and be confounded by the operation (unable to identify the cause of the bleeding). This series of 'events' have the potential to control how Radha's practice is actualised. I use the Deleuzian notion of 'event' here, where previously I had discussed 'event' as something that ruptures standard practice (Badiou 2005).

For Deleuze, an event is something that *dissolves* the subject: the individual and her parameters are *undone* by the 'new' which the event precipitates. For example, the series of events just outlined are implicated in how her practice is actualised – the guilt she feels over her daughter and the irritation she reports on being scolded by the medical director. These affective-emotive states could constitute a distraction or impediment to Radha fully engaging with the serious task ahead of her. Radha demonstrates good insight into how these aspects could detract from her very important goal to provide surgical care for the patient. She is aware of the impact of these 'emotional moments', as she calls it, without being fully cognisant of how exactly they may impact her thoughts and actions.

To apply this to Radha, her thoughts and actions contribute to producing an understanding or appreciation of the event which had not pre-existed her experience with the encounter. Earlier in the chapter I described how Radha had been advised during her training and had also heard stories about the 'importance of stopping' in surgery when all interventions were exhausted and proved futile. However, she had not truly appreciated this instruction until she found herself in that particular situation: 'virtual difference has the power to become in unforeseen ways, always more than this actual world and not limited by its already present flow', (Colebrook 2002, p. 96).

Surgical training has played a critical role in equipping Radha with the necessary skills of judgement and technical proficiency to bring order to the chaotic nature of emergency practice. However, what Radha has demonstrated in her thoughts and actions is the necessity for a particular pedagogic strategy that creates connections between transcendent knowledge and the immanence of real events of practice. Assimilated practices that overwhelm or totalise a surgeon's actions through a specific understanding of emergency surgery risk ignoring the 'local curations' (Atkinson 2011, chapter 9) of learning that occur in unanticipated events. What is demanded in such situations are pedagogic schemes that work alongside a learner's attempts to resolve or answer a particular problem.

3.8 How do surgeons (practitioners) emerge from the technical and practical complexities of training systems and complex practice?

In this final section to the chapter, I explore the ways in which the training structures and craft of surgery (procedural technical, practical knowledge and skill) can shape, influence and modulate the evolving surgeon professional. This exploration is conducted using some theories put forward by Gilbert Simondon (1924–1989), a French philosopher who wrote extensively on information, communication and technology. His work has only recently been translated into English text, reaching a far wider audience and influencing both Deleuze and Massumi who have been discussed in this book.

The expansion of technology and our increasing use of it in the modern world has been discussed critically within philosophy. Martin Heidegger (1977) wrote extensively on this subject. In brief, he viewed technological development as a distortion of how we ordered the world and understood it, including our cognitive perception of reality. He asserted that technology was alienating our sense of authenticity.

Simondon however, took a different view. He argued that the treatment of technology within philosophy was problematic because of society's efforts to judge novel technologies (e.g. in vitro fertilisation) through fixed and historic cultural values that are often irrelevant or 'behind the times' (Coombes 2012; Sauvagnargues 2012; Bardin 2015). This resonates with earlier arguments made by Deleuze who emphasized the challenges of transcendent frameworks when finding ways to embrace the immanence of events. I have chosen four key ideas that Simondon developed to support his argument and which have important implications for examining medical education and clinical training: *individuation, metastability, affect* and *hylomorphism*

Individuation

Simondon places emphasis on the *processes of becoming*, rather than on the already constituted individual ('being'). Individuation in simple terms relates to *how something emerges* and becomes constituted. He describes knowledge (epistemology) as grounded in a theory of *individuation* (how something emerges or becomes), meaning that it arises through the experience of an encounter in practice. This supports earlier arguments made as regards how subjects come to know something – the focus is not on what is known, but rather on the processes that constitute how knowledge is formed and developed: the individuation of knowledge. Simondon specifically emphasises *the conditions that determine what knowledge can be*: drawing attention to the relations, operations and interdependencies involved in the processes of becoming (Coombes 2012; Bardin 2015; Mills 2016).

Thus, as individuals, we are only ever partially formed, partially complete – we exist between serial processes of individuation, in a constant state of (re)forming between different modes of individuation (Scott 2014, p. 33). If we accept this premise, then learners and practitioners in medicine exist as *states of potential* continually undergoing processes of individuation through their encounters and experiences in the clinical world. An example is how Radha 'exists between individuations': in the encounter with the female patient, Radha describes her thoughts, emotions and actions as a mother, an employee of the NHS hospital, as a colleague, as an on-call surgeon, as a woman and as a fellow human being. These are all the different modes of individuation that form and develop as she encounters the different components of the clinical experience reflecting the various relations that she establishes in that same encounter. Appreciating the processes of individuation in a given moment draws attention to the variable factors that influence our thoughts and actions in an encounter of practice.

Metastability

Metastability (borrowed from thermodynamics) is the condition that makes individuation possible. It relates to states of tension which can be disrupted to release potentialities that can transform the learner or practitioner, leading to new or modified ontological states. Simondon uses the paradigm of crystallisation to help illustrate his ideas (Chabot 2003, pp. 79–84; Mills 2016, pp. 37–39). If a speck of dust disrupted a crystalline solution, crystals start to form. The crystalline solution is a metastable structure, it represents the many potentials of a learner/practitioner. Importantly, what is individuated is not just the crystal (for our purposes the learner or practitioner) but the crystal *in relation to its milieu*; an individual in relation to their potential or 'pool of becoming'. The notion of 'crystal in relation to its milieu' can be thought of as the learner engaging with the experience of the encounter.

We can draw parallels here with trainees in medicine and surgery. Each learner has the capacity to continually individuate and therefore she can have no fixed identity: this condition determines the nature of experience. Importantly, the potential to individuate resides in both the trainee as well as the relations the trainee forms within the encounter (milieu). For example, Radha individuates through the clinical encounter with the female patient, and her milieu (which comprises the environment she works in and the relations she forms within it) also individuates as the event unfolds.

> The individual, then, is always in relation to its milieu, which co-individuates along with it. As such the individual can never be considered as complete but always partial and in the process of individuation, the milieu always acting as a mediation between individual and world.
>
> (Mills 2016, p. 40)

The different states of potential in any encounter can never be completely exhausted ('used up') nor can they be entirely dissipated: for example, Radha's capacities in the situation she describes are limitless! A singularity – something(s) in a clinical event that disrupts our way of being – for example, Radha's inability to locate the bleeding point during the surgery acts to structure/individuate the potentials within that particular encounter. Through this process the encounter starts to become meaningful to the individual.

Affect

The important points to take away from Simondon's (1989) writings on affect are that, first, affect mediates individuation, that is, the processes of becoming. Second, affect emerges from the ways in which an individual orients herself when confronted by a disparity or tension in her environment. Put another way, affect arises from how the individual relates to herself as well as the environment it finds itself in.

To illustrate this concept I turn to a typical clinical scenario that many health-care professionals are all too familiar with. At the end of a morning outpatient clinic, an elderly patient, Mrs. Thurai, who is late for her clinic appointment, finally arrives, brought in by hospital transport. In this situation, the clinician is confronted by the encounter of a late yet elderly patient, which acts as the singularity, the speck of dust that transforms the crystalline milieu. The clinician responses (which emerges from a pool of potential ways to act, see or think) are initially mediated by affects that influence how the professional thinks, feel and eventually acts in this situation. Here are a sample of the factors which will impact the individuation of affective relations in this particular situation: the clinician is torn and irritated because clinic has overrun, he is late for an important radiology meeting, he has not eaten or drunk anything in hours and was expecting to grab a sandwich, there is no clinic room to see the patient as the rooms are being refreshed for the afternoon clinics, the consultation won't be quick because the elderly patient is physically immobile, partially sighted and deaf. These aspects of the encounter are also singularities which can in turn precipitate a myriad ways to think and act – an infinite state of potentials.

Thus, the subject in this situation is in a constant state of individuation mediated by affects that arise continually and reflect the relations the subject forms within the encounter from moment to moment and which indicate how the experience matters to the subject. Further, how the pool of potential ways to respond (the 'metastable system') operates in any encounter cannot be predicted because it is dependent on 'singularities', whereby each event can trigger a system of potentials that will actualise in ways that cannot be known in advance.

Hylomorphism

In Radha's narrative, as the interaction between herself and the patient unfolds and evolves, the potentialities that emerge from the encounter relate to her attempts to grasp the encounter, to make sense of what is happening. The encounter begins to take 'shape'. The potentialities that emerge and develop reflect the form or structure that is already present in the substance of the encounter. Thus, Simondon emphasizes that form is immanent to matter, which for my purposes means that any experience of learning or practice already has a structure within it, signified by the affective responses that emerge as the individual grapples with the event.

However, a hylomorphic framework signifies an external application of structure. An example is the didactic instruction on doctor-patient communication provided by *Good Medical Practice* (2013). This document details how Radha should interact and speak with the patient, through predefined notions of honesty, transparency and ethics. While it is advisable in complex situations to provide detailed guidance for a doctor to follow, this approach risks being ineffective if applied blindly to all situations. This is because it neglects to recognise how Radha has already encountered the situation, and how her prehension has informed the ways in which she decides to conduct herself in relation to the patient as well as to herself as a surgeon and fellow human being.

Simondon's theories illuminate the nature of the struggle that confronts clinicians and other healthcare professionals engaged in routine practice: that is, the tensions between the desires and values imposed upon the profession by the regulatory system (which in turn is set by society, national policy etc.) and the individual capacities that form and develop as a consequence of the potentials that arise from actual encounters of practice. However, what is often neglected by regulatory schemes is a recognition of the recurring causality between how practitioners view systems of regulation and how systems of regulation can alter the way practitioners think and act. In Chapters 4 and 5 I return to this theme.

3.9   Concluding thoughts

In this chapter I have developed a theoretical framework, a pedagogy of encounter, to understand and prioritise in the learning agenda *how something matters for a trainee*. This approach requires a softening of the transcendent frameworks that presently govern teaching practices and systems of training. It also raises issues of ethics within a pedagogic scenario, where ethics relates to the capacities to think and act which are brought to the fore by an engagement with a particular situation rather than the application of a broad moral code to practice.

The way in which a teacher understands something may be punctured by the trainee's response. An example from the procurement surgery narrative in the first chapter involves Vinny, the mentor surgeon, noticing the trainee's response. It appears that he had neither anticipated nor previously experienced such a reaction from a trainee. In this context an ethics of clinical pedagogies is concerned with conduct that is relative to a particular learning encounter, how it matters to the trainee and how the trainer engages with that trainee.

Through a pedagogy of encounter, I have explored relevant philosophical theories to illustrate how actual encounters of clinical experience can be analysed to illuminate the pedagogical opportunities embedded within. I have introduced a number of philosophers such as Alfred North Whitehead, Brian Massumi and Gilbert Simondon, who are gaining traction in wider spheres of education (school education, higher education, professional education) impacting pedagogic practices, but whose writings remain relatively understudied within clinical education and medical training, with limited application of their work.

I conclude with a passage from Susan Buck Morss (2010, p. 77), who comments on the narrow approach of traditional education systems and the unwillingness to contemplate the 'new' of a learner's experience and practice because this may not fit the parameters of what is known and accepted. Pedagogies of encounter are less concerned with inducting learners into existing bodies of knowledge and prioritise instead the infinite ways in which they learn and come to know things. Developing and promoting such strategies within medical education is to configure learning in clinical environments as an adventure, where the outcome is uncertain and the modes of becoming unknown yet soon to be.

> There is a blindness to institutionalised education that passes down the authority of tradition, a mental timidity, born of privilege or just plain laziness, that cloaks itself in the heavy bombast of cultural heritage and historic preservation. It generates enormous resistance to trespassing conceptual boundaries or exceeding the limits of present imagination, rewarding instead the virtues of scholastic diligence, disciplinary professionalism and elitist erudition, all escape routes from the pragmatic necessity of confronting the new. Indeed extreme discomfort is caused by the truly new, the truly 'contemporary', that which Nietzsche called the 'untimely' – those aspects of the present moment that simply do not fit our established traditions or modes of understanding.

References

Atkinson, D. (2011). *Art, Equality and Learning: Pedagogies Against the State*. Rotterdam, Boston, Taipei: Sense Publishers.

Atkinson, D. (2016). "Without Criteria: Art and Learning and the Adventure of Pedagogy." *International Journal of Art and Design Education*. doi:10.1111/jade.12089.

Atkinson, D. (2018). *Art, Disobedience and Ethics: The Adventure of Pedagogy*. Palgrave Macmillan.

Badiou, A. (2005). *Being and Event*. London and New York: Continuum.

Barad, K. (2007). *Meeting the Universe Halfway: Quantum Physics and the Entanglement of Matter and Meaning*. Duke University Press.

Bardin, A. (2015). *Epistemology and Political Philosophy in Gilbert Simondon: Individuation, Technics, Social Systems*. London and New York: Springer.

Bordage, G. (2009). "Conceptual Frameworks to Illuminate and Magnify." *Medical Education*, 43: 312–319.

Buch, A., and Andersen, V. (2015). "Team and Project Work in Engineering Practices." *Nordic Journal of Working Life Studies*, 5 (3): 27–46.

Buck-Morss, S. (2010). "The Second Time as Farce . . . Historical Pragmatics and the Untimely Present." In Douzinas, C., and Zizek, S. (Eds.), *The Idea of Communism* (pp. 67–80). London and New York: Verso.

Chabot, P. (2003). The Philosophy of Simondon, trans by Krefetz, A. and Kirkpatrick, G. Bloomsbury Academic.

Colebrook, C. (2002). Gilles Deleuze. London & New York: Routledge.

Coombes, M. (2012). *Gilbert Simondon and the Philosophy of the Transindividual*, trans. LaMarre, T. Boston: MIT Press.

Dall Jensen, R., Syer-Hansen, M., et al. (2018). "Being a Surgeon or Doing Surgery? A Qualitative Study of Learning in the Operating Room." *Medical Education*, 52: 861–876.

Deleuze, G. (1994). *Difference and Repetition*, trans. Patton, P. Continuum.

Deleuze, G., and Guattari, F. (1977). *Anti-Oedipus*, trans. Hurley, R., Seem, M., and Lane, H. New York: Viking.

Deleuze, G. and Guattari, F. (2004). A Thousand Plateaus: Capitalism and Schizophrenia. New York/London: Continuum.

Ericsson, K. A., Krampe, R. T., and Tesch-Romer, C. (1993). "The Role of Deliberate Practice in the Acquisition of Expert Performance." *Psychological Review*, 100 (3): 363–406.

Fenwick, T. (2014). "Sociomateriality in Medical Practice and Learning: Attuning to What Matters." *Medical Education*, 48: 44–52.

General Medical Council. (2016). *Promoting Excellence: Standards for Medical Education and Training*. Retrieved from www.gmc-uk.org/Promoting_excellence_standards_for_medical_education_and_training_0715.pdf_61939165.pdf.

Gillespie, H., Kelly, M., et al. (2018). "How Can Tomorrow's Doctors Be More Caring? A Phenomenological Investigation." *Medical Education*, 52: 1052–1063.

Greenhalgh, T. (2013). "Uncertain and Clinical Method." In Somers, L., and Launer, J. (Eds.), *Clinical Uncertainty in Primary Care: The Challenge of Collaborative Engagement*. New York: Springer.

Greenhalgh, T. (2014). "Evidence-Based Medicine: A Movement in Crises?" *British Medical Journal*, 348: g3725.

Guenter, D., Fowler, N., and Lee, L. (2011). "Clinical Uncertainty: Helping Our Learners." *Canadian Family Physician*, 57 (1): 120–122.

Heidegger, M. (1977). Question Concerning Technology and Other Essays. New York: Harper Perennial.

Intercollegiate Surgical Curriculum (ISC). (2016). *The Intercollegiate Surgical Curriculum for General Surgery*. Retrieved from www.iscp.ac.uk/curriculum/surgical/spe cialty_year_syllabus.aspx?enc=Ttek+oCN/eOTQZ3fsf5KIg==.

Kemmis, S., Wilkinson, J., Edwards-Groves, C., et al. (2014). *Changing Practices, Changing Education*. London: Springer.

Kolb, D. (1984). *Experiential Learning*. Englewood Cliffs, NJ: Prentice Hall.

Lave, J., and Wenger, E. (1991). *Situated Learning. Legitimate Peripheral Participation*. New York: Cambridge University Press.

Logan, R. L., and Scott, P. J. (1996). "Uncertainty in Clinical Practice: Implications for Quality and Costs of Health Care." *Lancet*, 347 (9001): 595–598.

Massumi, B. (2002). *Parables for the Virtual*. Durham, NC: Duke University Press.

McConnell, M. M., and Eva, K. W. (2012). "The Role of Emotion in the Learning and Transfer of Clinical Skills and Knowledge." *Academic Medicine*, 87 (10): 1316–1322.

McNaughton, N. (2013). "Discourse(s) of Emotion Within Medical Education: The Ever-Present Absence." *Medical Education*, 47 (1): 71–79.

Mills, S. (2016). *Gilbert Simondon: Information, Technology and Media*. London and New York: Rowman & Littlefield.

Phillips, A. W., and Jones, A. E. (2015). "The Validity and Reliability of Workplace Based Assessments in Surgical Training." *The Bulletin*, 97 (3): e19–e23.

Phillips, A. W., Lim, J., et al. (2016). "Case-Based Discussions: UK Surgical Trainee Perceptions." *Clinical Teacher*, 13 (3): 207–212.

Polanyi, M. (1958). *Personal Knowledge: Towards a Post-Critical Philosophy*. Chicago, IL: University of Chicago Press.

Polanyi, M. (2009). *The Tacit Dimension*. Chicago, IL: University of Chicago Press.

Royal College of Surgeons of England. (2014). *Good Surgical Practice*. RCSE: Professional Standards.

Sackett, D. L., Rosenberg, W. M. C., et al. (1996). "Evidence Based Medicine: What It Is and What It Isn't." *British Medical Journal*, 312 (7023): 71–72.

Sauvagnargues, A. (2012). Crystals and Membranes: Individuation and Temporality. Trans. J. Roffe. In Gilbert Simondon. Being and Technology, A. De Boever, A. Murray, J. Roffe and A. Woodward eds.: 57–70. Edinburgh: Edinburgh University Press.

Schon, D. A. (1983). *The Reflective Practitioner*. London: Temple Smith.

Scott, D. (2014). Gilbert Simondon's Psychic and Collective Individuation: A Critical Introduction and Guide. Edinburgh: Edinburgh University Press.

Shaviro, S. (2012). *Without Criteria: Kant, Whitehead, Deleuze and Aesthetics*. MIT Press.

Simondon, G. (1989). *Individuation Psychique et Collective*. Paris: Aubier.

Spinoza, B. (1996). *Ethics*. London: Penguin.

Timmermans, S., and Berg, M. (2003). *The Gold Standard: The Challenge of Evidence-Based Medicine and Standardisation in Health Care*. Philadelphia: Temple University Press.

Vygotsky, L. (1978). *The Mind in Society – Development of Higher Psychological Processes*. Cambridge: Harvard University Press.

West, A. F., and West, R. R. (2002). "Clinical Decision-Making: Coping with Uncertainty." *Postgraduate Medical Journal*, 78: 319–321.

Whitehead, A. N. (1929). *Process and Reality*. New York: The Free Press.

Yuill, C., Crinson, I., and Duncan, E. (2010). *Key Concepts in Health Studies*. London: Sage Publications Ltd.

Part II

Representations of Clinical Practice

ideologies, complexities and candour

4 Conceptions of Care and Caring

complicated procedures versus
complex experiences

Every day, doctors and other healthcare professionals engage with the public within different clinical scenarios and medical environments but always with the same aim – to provide an individual with the necessary and appropriate 'care'. Within modern clinical practice, 'care' is conceptualised beyond the provision of cure, remedy or treatment. The concept of care and caring has been theorised, analysed, debated and written about from a number of perspectives. The exhaustive literature on the topic, primarily from the nursing profession, examines the different theories of caring (Leininger 2001; Watson 2008; Roache 1997), what should constitute the fundamental components of care (Kitson et al. 2010, 2016), the notion of compassionate care (Kret 2011; Papadopoulos et al. 2015) and the development of elder care and palliative care (van der Cingel 2011; Bradley et al. 2001). In the last decade person-centred care has emerged as a framework to direct and develop the approach and services available for those seeking medical care (Health Foundation 2016). In essence, it focuses on the needs of the individual rather than on the priorities of the service, so that a person's (the patient) preferences, values and beliefs drive the ways in which they are cared for and treated.

In this chapter, the notion of care is extended to consider the emerging *relations* that form and develop through the physician *responding* to the concerns of a patient about their mental or physical health. In particular, what is explored is the *nature of the encounter* between patient and doctor: *complex* layers of relations interweaving with *complicated* medical processes. What does this mean? The following ethnographic account illustrates how the inherent uncertainty of medical practice can give rise to the development of different forms or ideologies of care to emerge *within*, *through* and *from* clinical encounters.

The giving and receiving of care as experienced respectively by patients (receivers of care) and doctors ('givers' of care) is characterised by human interactions suffused with affect, emotion and challenging communication. This is established, here, as differentiated from a patient's plan of care which comprises the multiple complicated processes of theoretical and technical details, estimations of adverse events or risk and procedural logistics. I have identified the latter as Official Care to emphasize how these forms of care arise from formal clinical guidelines and professional documents and are, in turn, enacted by the subjects of these texts (patients and doctors). Whilst the former concerns actual experiences of care that

I refer to as *Real Care* (the 'real' denotes the reality of undergoing a process of care and the resulting experience).

The use of the descriptors 'Real' and 'Official' is adapted from Ian Stronach's (2010) analysis of how teenage pregnancy in the modern era has been framed in the public domain (p. 46). These two ideologies of care can overlap as well as diverge in an encounter of practice. The tension and conflict that can arise between these different forms of care is the main exploration of this chapter.

Through the central concept of surgical care, I investigate the difference between how to give appropriate care in unanticipated or unpredictable clinical situations, and how care is treated as a major concept (defined, developed and framed) within professional texts and clinical guidelines. Certain relevant and impactful texts are analysed to locate key themes and concepts around the 'giving' of care. Information presented in these texts have helped shape education and training practices in the United Kingdom. Such texts include *Good Medical Practice (2013)*, the GMC published guidance and other texts on professional values and conduct. In the following chapter, how professional guidance is enacted in unanticipated events of real practice is explored.

The Art of Care

"Oh hello, this is Arundathi, one of the transplant doctors. I just wanted to see if Dr. Chou was available to discuss how Mr. Pitt's procedure is progressing?" I settle into my chair, knowing that it could be as long as ten minutes before someone picks up the phone and comes back to me with an answer. However, my effort at getting comfy has been premature; within seconds I hear the receiver click (what a pleasant surprise!), "Mr. Pitt is . . .," the words are drowned out by an approaching trolley being wheeled onto the ward. I peer into the trolley. The occupier is Mr. Pitt (who should still be in the procedure room!). I return to my phone call and say wearily, "Mr. Pitt didn't have the procedure did he? I mean . . . I know Dr. Chou is one of the best, but even he couldn't have got a stent in that quickly." The voice on the other end is Dr. Chou. "Hi Arundi, your gentleman refused to have the procedure, not much I can do I'm afraid. Come back to me when he agrees."

Dr. Chou is probably my favourite radiologist. A calm demeanour and friendly manner belie an impressive skill set. He is notoriously polite to patients and colleagues alike. Therefore, I am puzzled as to why my patient is back on the ward, sans procedure.

Mr. Pitt is now happily ensconced in his bed, patient bay 4. He catches my eye as I approach his bed. "Hello love, I did as you said but when I got there that fella was terrifying! So they sent me back up." "But Mr. Pitt, they told me that you refused to have the procedure. Why did you do that? We talked about it last night and I explained to you that the tube connecting your kidney to your bladder has got a narrowing in it, which means the urine made by your kidney can't reach your bladder. Do you remember the picture I drew? Where

I showed you how your kidney is starting to resemble a balloon because of all that urine backed up and trapped in the kidney, blowing it up? That's why you haven't been able to pee, because there's a blockage in that tube. Dr. Chou was going to relieve that block by placing a stent in the tube so that the urine could flow into your bladder again. It means you'll be able to pee again."

Mr. Pitt turns to the side table and opens the drawer pulling out a sheet of paper with my drawing from the previous night. "I know what you said love, but that chappy (Dr. Chou) told me I had to sign a consent form so he could do the procedure and then he told me that there was a chance the stent could make a hole in my kidney . . . 50% or something . . . then I'd lose my kidney . . . I can't go back on dialysis again . . . I just can't . . ." He looks at me, utterly devastated and terrified. I walk to his bedside and sit with him. "It's ok," I say soothingly but he has seen my disappointment and exasperation, I cannot hide it this morning. He clenches my palm between his bony fingers. This day has left him bewildered, tired and now he feels guilty.

"The chances of something like that happening . . . I think Dr. Chou would have called it a rupture or perforation, well it's rare . . . he possibly quoted a percentage to you, and I know that I wasn't there, but I can assure you that it wouldn't have been as high as 50%," I continue. "We wouldn't recommend the procedure unless the risk was so small (I pinch my finger and thumb together in a physical demonstration of 'smallness') that it was acceptable for you to go through with it . . . you see at this moment the risk of the procedure going wrong is tiny, in fact it's much, much smaller than the risk of your kidney being damaged by the blockage." "But he didn't say that," he says, dejected. "He said I'd sure as lose it (the kidney)!"

4.1   Real care

This account perfectly illustrates some of the issues around patient care that led to the desire for a person-centred care movement. Kidney transplant and dialysis patients live with chronic conditions that require ongoing clinical surveillance and support. This experience is frequently exhausting, demoralising and often leaves the patient feeling disengaged and disempowered from important decision-making processes about their medical care. The literature on person-centred care draws attention to the importance of 'meaningful participation' and shared decision-making (Cribb and Entwistle 2011; Epstein and Street 2011). However, despite raising awareness and making efforts to power share, the reality is that a hierarchy of relationships form around different levels of engagement, responsibility and shared goals (Wolf et al. 2017). The result is a spectrum of involvement which ranges from participation at the lowest level to partnership at the highest level (Frank et al 2009). These issues around partnership are certainly illustrated in this short encounter between Mr. Pitt, myself and Dr. Chou. However, in this chapter I want to move beyond a discussion on the dynamics of power to focus on the *affective relations* that form and develop between patient and doctor in situations of *uncertain* medical encounters.

In particular, the narrative depicts the *typologies* of *Real Care*: the sub-categories of care that constitute a patient's everyday experience. These include *care as experienced by the patient*, for example on the ward, during the diagnostic process, in the radiology suite and through encounters with two doctors. It also comprises the *experience of providing care* on the part of the two doctors and other personnel involved in Mr. Pitt's inpatient stay. Each category of Real Care is subject to two agendas: the intended provision of care (the plan of care devised by the professional team responsible for diagnosis and treatment) and the actual experience of care (the patient's physical, psychological, emotional and cognitive perceptions of care, as well as the impressions of the physicians 'doing' the care-giving). In this specific instance, the intended provision of care was the treatment (i.e. insertion of a stent) decided upon by myself and Dr. Chou. However, the actual experience of care by the patient undergoing this treatment was fear, bewilderment, guilt and a risk of acting foolishly. Dr. Chou assured me afterwards that he had not quoted a complication risk of 50%, whereas Mr. Pitt insisted that he had heard exactly that figure when being advised of the risk of losing his kidney. I believe them both.

It is clear that Mr. Pitt was desperate to salvage his kidney transplant yet deterred by something. Was he suddenly frightened at the dawning realisation of the procedure? Did the risk appear more exaggerated to him? Did Dr. Chou fail to engage with the patient in a manner appropriate to soothe Mr. Pitt's doubts and fears? It is also possible that factors that neither Dr. Chou nor I had anticipated were responsible for Mr. Pitt's refusal to go through with the procedure. My experience of providing care for Mr. Pitt was one of disappointment and frustration with both the system and my colleague. Equally, Dr. Chou may have been dissatisfied and worried that a patient who required an urgent procedure failed to receive it. As this narrative demonstrates, an event of patient care in actual clinical practice (Real Care) is composed of multiple layers, each concealing hidden complexity and nuance, which inevitably contribute further to the *contingent* nature of care.

Experiences of care cannot ever be fully predicted or foreseen. Adherence to clinical guidelines may improve the clinical outcome for the patient by removing some of the uncertainty and, thereby, potentially enhancing a patient's experience of care. But it cannot completely control the *quality* of the experience or the *manner* in which it is experienced. The term 'experience' is used in this chapter to describe *how a person encounters something*, that is, how she perceives, discerns or happens upon an event, person or object, as well as what impressions this leaves upon her. Certainly, the format of a procedure (here, radiological insertion of stent), the theoretical knowledge underlying a diagnosis (here, an obstructed kidney due to a narrowing in the outflow tube [ureter]) and the remedy for a clinical problem may be common knowledge and form habitual practice. Nonetheless, how a plan of care is fully experienced, as well as what may unfold in that experiencing, is always an unknown. Therefore, notions of Real Care are grounded in the uncertainty or *contingency of actual practice*. This uncertainty determines *how* a form of care is experienced, as a temporal reality (over time).

The impact of uncertainty on skill perception

The literature on uncertainty, as discussed in the previous chapter, tends towards examining the phenomenon as it arises through the elements of clinical competence, namely, processes of diagnosis, clinical decision-making and medical judgement (Latifi et al. 2013; Pauley et al. 2011; Jalote-Parmar and Badke-Schaub 2008; Sutton et al. 2015; Flin et al. 2007). Logan and Scott (1996) attribute uncertainty in health care partly to the imprecision inherent in decision-making. Guenter et al. (2011) describe how, in contingent situations, trainees experience effort and anxiety in 'maintaining a cloak of competence' (p. 120). This refers to the spectrum of emotions experienced by trainees when their practice is challenged by the uncertainty that arises due to unfamiliarity, limitations in skill or an inability to meet patient expectations

Professional documents that focus on the fluency of a surgeon's practice, as defined by those elements of performance that can be *measured* directly (e.g. technical skills, behaviours and attitudes, theoretical knowledge) demonstrate a belief that ensuring proficiency in these aspects of skills training is the primary solution to eliminating the unpredictability of practice. Certainly, developing fluent skill in the component parts of a procedure is critical in the effort to ensure that patients come to no harm and benefit from successful interventions. An example is the DOPS (direct observation of procedural skill) evaluation, which forms a core part of trainee assessment in the formative years of training (see Chapter 7 where examples of assessment tools are critically analysed).

A consequence to this process is that skills that can be measured directly, and, by virtue of this fact become '*visible*' to the world, are prioritised (by the curriculum), recognised (by training practices) and resultantly representative of what it means to be a competent doctor. In turn, this engenders a belief that orienting training around aspects of measurable and visible performance will reduce uncertainty in practice or eliminate the sources of error associated with practice. For example, my inability to participate in the procurement (because I was speechless and physically paralysed by the reality of the event of practice) may be attributed to failed practice owing to a lack of exposure: 'there'll be a next time . . . you just need to do more, that's all' (Vinny's comments). This evaluation reveals the widespread belief held by surgeons and consolidated by educational documents (e.g. curriculae, operative manuals) that repetitive, technical practice and recurrent exposure to events will, in and of themselves, minimise the variability of experiences 'in the field'. It follows therefore that repeated experience will strengthen a surgeon's capacity to respond.

There is no doubt that repetitive practice and the accumulation of experience are critical to developing a surgeon's ability, confidence and safe practice. However, the difficulty arises when, despite the best preparations, a clinical encounter can culminate in unanticipated and unpredictable outcomes. In spite of the uncertainty intrinsic to most, if not all, clinical encounters, these instances can be perceived as tantamount to an *error in practice*, constituted by a lack of experience or failure in judgement or skill. I would add that the single-minded pursuit of eliminating error from clinical events obscures what should always be the primary objective of medical practice and the purpose of training: providing care for the patient and learning how to care for the patient, respectively, in all manner of circumstances. In the earlier narrative, the goal of Mr. Pitt's clinical encounter was not accomplished – he did not receive the necessary care. No stent was placed to relieve the obstruction in his failing kidney transplant. The patient was left confused, distressed and guilt-ridden, whilst the doctors were left both frustrated in their attempts to provide urgent care and anxious about the wellbeing of their patient.

Providing certainty in the face of contingency

I suggest that it is at this interface of Real Care – the unpredictable nature of a clinical encounter – that the role of the doctor is constructed for the patient in an enduring and forceful manner. In a world that is increasingly technologized, in part to detach from the human propensity for error, the value and professional longevity of a doctor may lie in how she mediates the contingency of clinical practice to give patients much-needed reassurance and comfort. If a doctor is successful in this endeavour, then she may paradoxically give patients that elusive factor: a sense of certainty in their medical care.

> The current attempt to extinguish uncertainty in our society risks removing from the medical profession some important 'tools of the trade' and placing obstacles in their way. Too much emphasis in medical training on removing or reducing uncertainty will crowd out what little attention is being paid to educating doctors into the maturity and wisdom that they require to be able to accompany people in times of need, contain their own and their patients' anxieties and facilitate healing and recovery in an uncertain world.
>
> (West and West 2002, p. 320)

4.2   Official care

What is the purpose of examining how care is conceived and deployed in professional texts or policy documents? What does such an investigation tell us? It provides critical insights into and background on how guidance on patient care is enacted in actual clinical practice. This has significant implications for exploring how clinicians and trainees experience events of medical (e.g. surgical) practice. This analytical approach borrows from Michel Foucault's method of historical analysis, which he called 'genealogy': 'a form of history that can account for the constitution of knowledges, discourses, domains of objects and so on, without having to make reference to a subject that is either transcendental in relation to the field of events or runs in its empty sameness throughout the course of history' (Faubion 2002, p. 118). Instead of examining phenomena from a linear perspective (i.e. start at the past and work towards the present), Foucault examines the practices and discourses that constitute the subject of study. In this particular case I explore how the professional identity and practices of trainees/surgeons are constituted in policy discourses, what the conditions are under which statements about training practices are formed at a given time, whose voice is privileged in the discourses (i.e. whose interest does such a conception of care serve?) and which voices are silent.

By looking at the practices, institutions and discourses that constitute how patient care is conceived, developed and delivered, one can then begin to explore questions regarding the objectives and aims of policies regarding medical training and clinical education.

The formal discourses on how doctors are trained to provide care are created by the stakeholders in medical education policy. These stakeholders include the General Medical Council (GMC), the Academic Medical Colleges (e.g. the Royal College of Physicians and the Royal College of Surgeons), postgraduate medical deaneries, NHS Employers (NHSE), Health Education England and the Department of Health. Meanwhile, *Good Medical Practice* (General Medical Council 1995, 1998, 2001, 2006, 2013), which I abbreviate to *GMP* (see Figures 4.1 and 4.2), can be considered the primary text which provides both a framework for how doctors should organize and structure their practice and also guidance on how doctors should conduct themselves as caregivers. *GMP* is written by the GMC, who are responsible for licensing medical practitioners. The GMC is also responsible for setting the duties and responsibilities of a doctor in the United Kingdom, setting the standards of training programs, conceiving the processes for assessment and formulating the professional requirements for maintaining licensure (GMC 1993, 2016). To provide a historical context and rationale for the structure and content of *GMP* (2013), I examined Department of Health policy texts published around the same time period. In 2014, the Royal Colleges of Surgeons of England published a related text that adapted the principles and guidance set out in *GMP* for the surgical profession. *Good Surgical Practice* (Royal College of Surgeons of England [RCS] 2014), which I abbreviate to *GSP*, presented specific guidance for surgeons engaged in surgical practice. Before proceeding to a discussion of the text itself, it is prudent at this point to briefly look at the organisation that is the GMC in order to understand its role and standing amongst the medical profession.

Good Medical Practice (GMP)

GMP was first published in 1995 by the GMC to replace existing guidance on unacceptable behaviour in the medical profession, specifically that which would lead to a charge of professional misconduct at a disciplinary hearing of the GMC.[1]

> It was a kind of handbook for 'doctors in trouble', you know, you had been found negligent or had harmed a patient in some way, and this booklet basically told you what you shouldn't do. It was pretty obvious stuff, like 'don't be rude to your patients'. Things like that. Hardly rocket science!
>
> (Stephen, Consultant Surgeon)

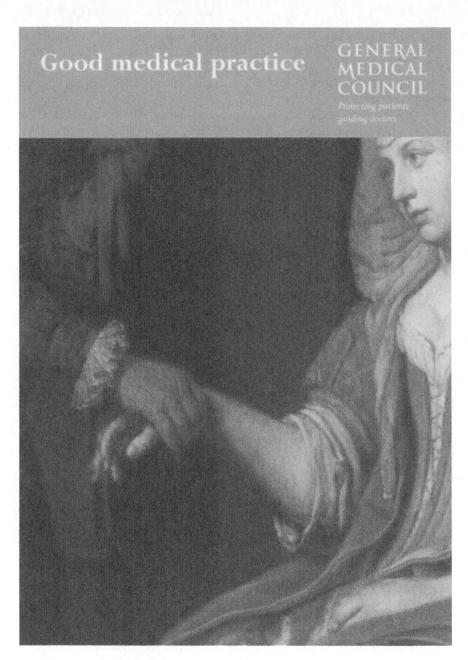

Figure 4.1 Cover image of *Good Medical Practice* (1995).

Source: Copyright General Medical Council, reproduced with permission.

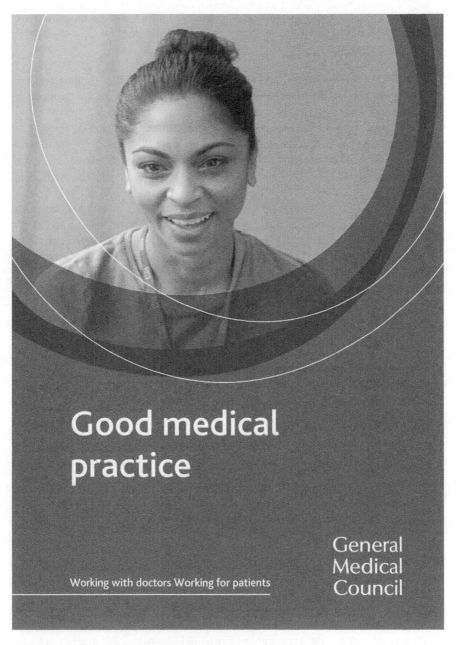

Figure 4.2 Cover image of *Good Medical Practice* (2013).

Source: Copyright General Medical Council, reproduced with permission.

With the approaching spectre of appraisal and revalidation for doctors, the GMC overhauled the document in 2005 with the aim of circulating it as a handbook for all doctors in practice.

> The 2005/6 review considered the approach to giving guidance: that it should focus on good practice rather than list 'offences'; that it should apply to all doctors on the register; that it should establish principles and standards rather than specify particular requirements or prohibitions. We do not propose to re-open these issues in this review, although we will of course respond positively if the issues are raised by other organisations or individuals.
>
> (GMC 2010, p. 3)

Picker Europe (2006) were commissioned by the GMC to conduct research amongst doctors, patients and the public. Their aim was to look at 'what are the key duties of a doctor for inclusion in *Good Medical Practice*; the balance between the roles of patients, doctors and other health professionals; the balance between clinical and organisational duties; and whether or not it is reasonable to expect doctors to adhere to all duties all the time' (Picker Europe 2006, p. 1).

GMP was most recently updated and re-released in 2013. It categorises a doctor's practice into four component areas, or, domains (GMC 2013):

- Domain 1: knowledge, skills and performance
- Domain 2: safety and quality
- Domain 3: communication, partnership and teamwork
- Domain 4: maintaining trust

Figure 4.3 illustrates the list of criteria that constitute each domain and which every doctor must comply with in order to meet the standards of that specific subcategory of practice.

4.3   How is care represented in *GMP* (1995) in contrast to *GMP* (2013)?

In the intervening years between the two publications, how has the notion of care transformed?

Imagery

The front cover of the 1995 text depicts a Michael Van Musscher portrait, 'Doctor taking a young woman's pulse' (see Figure 4.1). The pale, feminine hand is held purposefully by a male doctor. This image portrays the doctor as self-appointed protector, guardian and expert bearer of scientific knowledge, whilst the patient is female, passive, submissive and the object of the physician's benevolence and expert knowledge. It illustrates the dominance of paternalism in that era, which

Contents

Figure 4.3 Contents page of *GMP* (2013).

Source: Copyright General Medical Council, reproduced with permission.

prevailed in constructions of the doctor-patient relationship. There is a large body of literature exploring paternalism in clinical practice (Dworkin 1992; McKinstry 1992; O'Neill 1984; Siegler 1985), which I will not replicate here. More pointedly, the use of this image in a doctor's guidebook suggests that the established face of care in 1995 was informed by a paternalistic model of medicine. This theme is continued in the epithet featured beneath the GMC logo, 'Protecting patients guiding doctors'. It declares the dual roles of the organisation as self-appointed 'protector' and 'guide.'

In contrast, the covering image on the most recent publication of *GMP* (2013) (See Figure 4.2) bears the sole image of a young female doctor from an ethnic minority background. She is smiling broadly, and she appears engaged and happy at work. Such is an intended reflection of the diversity and increasingly female population of the medical workforce. Presumably the use of a cheery, youthful image presents the modern face of clinical medicine that many patients are likely to encounter – approachable, amiable, receptive and compassionate clinicians. The epithet beneath the logo now reads, 'working with doctors working for patients'. This modification of the organisational motto reflects a change in the philosophy of both the GMC and clinical medicine in the millennium: from paternalism to partnership. The organisation now promotes an egalitarian approach to the way in which it conceives caregivers (doctors) and recipients of care (patients). It works alongside doctors in a supportive and advisory capacity, guiding their practices of care whilst also engaging with patients through advocacy to ensure that their needs are voiced and met satisfactorily. Today, the doctor does not occupy the omnipotence of the first image. Rather, she is subject to the power of inspection and audit, processes introduced, in part, to prioritise the clinical care and safety of the patient as well as to improve the patient experience. The contrasting imagery emphasizes the change in the *locus of power* within the doctor-patient care relationship.

The 'good doctor'

In the opening pages of *GMP* (2013, p. a2) the following statement is made:

> Patients must be able to trust doctors with their lives and health. To justify that trust you must show respect for human life and make sure your practice meets the standards expected of you in four domains.

Life and health are perceived through a lens of disease and treatment, constituting the patient as a medical object. It proceeds to introduce the notion of the 'good doctor':

> Patients need good doctors. Good doctors make the care of their patients their first concern: they are competent, keep their knowledge and skills up to date, establish and maintain good relationships with patients and colleagues, are honest and trustworthy, and act with integrity and within the law.

> Good doctors work in partnership with patients and respect their rights to privacy and dignity. They treat each patient as an individual. They do their best to make sure all patients receive good care and treatment that will support them to live as well as possible, whatever their illness or disability.
>
> (ibid., 4)

There is an expansive body of research devoted to what constitutes a 'good doctor', and also to how a 'good doctor' is perceived (Corrado 2011; Judge and Solomon 1993; Jung et al. 1998). The symbolic evocation of the term 'good doctor' as virtuous and demonstrating 'goodness' deserves some discussion here. Within the pages of *GMP* the 'goodness' of the doctor is conceived through a set of practical criteria that must be achieved by a clinician for her to be recognised as a 'good doctor' by the GMC, which acts in its capacity, here, as a professional regulator and licensing authority. The framework outlines that a 'good doctor' should 'make the care of their patients their first concern'. This is through accomplishing proficiency in their work, in demonstrating their knowledge and skills as current and in exhibiting good interpersonal skills, honesty and integrity. These criteria reference the elements of performance that make up the four domains of practice upon which assessments, appraisal and revalidation are based. Deconstructing the 'goodness' of the 'good doctor' into these component parts may facilitate ease of assessment of performance and thus meet the surveillance and regulatory functions of the GMC. But do these criteria adequately capture the contingency of a doctor's practice or the full complexities of good clinical care? I don't believe they do. I suggest this reductive attempt to define and encapsulate how a doctor *cares* for her patients supports a current criticism of medical practice as a 'tick box exercise' (Cleland et al. 2014).

In the narrative of Mr. Pitt, two competent doctors (Dr. Chou and myself) with the patient's best interests at heart failed to deliver appropriate care. Did the procedure fail to occur because of a problem in communication skills? Certainly, communication appears to be problematic in this clinical encounter, though all parties attempted to be clear and transparent. Without diminishing the importance of good communication, I want to draw attention to other issues, separate to communication, which may feature in why the plan of care failed. There were a number of steps that constituted the care plan for this patient. All these steps were achieved, namely, the correct diagnosis and treatment plan was designed, up-to-date knowledge and skill were demonstrated (i.e. stent was inserted by the most experienced radiologist in the department) and doctors involved in patient care communicated appropriately to expedite an urgent procedure. In this conception of practice, care is viewed as a *complicated* procedural event, that is, the culmination of a series of complicated steps identified as indicative of good clinical care.

However, as discussed earlier, *Real Care* – the concrete experience of providing and receiving care – relates to the *complexities* of actual clinical practice, wherein the reality of care unfolds in everyday clinical encounters or through the *haecceities* of practice. In this conception of care, as already seen, the *force of affect* emerges within medical encounters in ways that can neither be predicted nor foreseen. The affective force of encounters exceeds the expected effects of rational behaviour. For example, in the case of Mr. Pitt, the affect that formed and developed when he interpreted the doctor's words through a growing anxiety impacted subsequent thoughts and actions in ways that could not have been anticipated fully. I suggest that negotiating the tension between care as a sequence of *complicated steps* versus care as contingent *complex practice* is the crux of how to be a 'good doctor'.

4.3   Complicated steps versus complex practice

The content of material between the two editions of *GMP* (1995, 2013) has not altered greatly. This may seem surprising given that *GMP* (1995) was a guide for failing doctors and, as such, the content was originally written to provide clear instructions for doctors who were struggling to meet the basic requirements of patient care. The recent publication (GMP 2013) has kept the original material but has altered the layout of the content; it is presented through a bullet-point format and also in a series of paragraphs. This arrangement is consistent with a conception and presentation of care as a sequence of (complicated) steps that must be enacted (outlined earlier). An example is the excerpt here, taken from the domain entitled 'Knowledge, Skills & Performance' (GMP 2013, p. 8), in which care is broken down into and explained through its prescriptive component parts.

Underneath each subheading of care there are a number of items that comprise attitudes or behaviours that a clinician must demonstrate to complete the necessary criteria. The danger inherent within this approach is that these criteria can distract the focus of the clinical encounter away from an engagement with the

16   In providing clinical care you must:

a   prescribe drugs or treatment, including repeat prescriptions, only when you have adequate knowledge of the patient's health and are satisfied that the drugs or treatment serve the patient's needs[6]
b   provide effective treatments based on the best available evidence
c   take all possible steps to alleviate pain and distress whether or not a cure may be possible[7]
d   consult colleagues where appropriate
e   respect the patient's right to seek a second opinion
f   check that the care or treatment you provide for each patient is compatible with any other treatments the patient is receiving, including (where possible) self-prescribed over-the-counter medications
g   wherever possible, avoid providing medical care to yourself or anyone with whom you have a close personal relationship.[6]

Figure 4.4 Good clinical care.

Source: (GMP 2013, p. 8) Copyright General Medical Council, reproduced with permission.

patient as and when indicated, to a preoccupation with meeting authorised criteria. This places an emphasis on the *process* of care rather than on *what actually happens* and *what is experienced* at each stage of care. Figure 4.4 constitutes care in simple, mechanistic terms that in no way reflect the complexities of doctor-patient relations. Nor does it reflect all the intensities that affect such relations or how a doctor might cope with the situation, as illustrated by the opening narrative. To return to the story of Mr. Pitt, whilst the steps in the process of care were accomplished, the objective of the care plan was not.

Figure 4.5 comprises an excerpt from Domain 4, where instructions on how to 'act with honesty and integrity' (ibid., 21) are issued. The requirements made of the doctor are didactic and specific. Handbooks providing guidance are useful precisely because they act as a point of reference, that is, a source that can be delved into at times of uncertainty, or when there is a query. The challenge, however, is to provide guidance and advice as opposed to rigidly enforce a written code of conduct. But, as seen in Figure 4.5, instructions on conduct are organised as a series of paragraphs and points, suggestive of a regulatory code of conduct and reminiscent of the style of a legal statute. The 'legalification' of non-legal fields is a pervading feature in this and *Good Surgical Practice* (2014). 'Legalification' is a term I use to connote when non-legal documents are structured in ways that resemble legal statutes and other contractual documents used in legislation and systems of law.

There is a growing trend towards legalification in other aspects of work and life; schools, universities, offices and other places of work have increasingly

Act with honesty and integrity

Honesty

65 You must make sure that your conduct justifies your patients' trust in you and the public's trust in the profession.
66 You must always be honest about your experience, qualifications and current role.
67 You must act with honesty and integrity when designing, organising or carrying out research, and follow national research governance guidelines and our guidance.[2]

Communicating information

68 You must be honest and trustworthy in all your communication with patients and colleagues. This means you must make clear the limits of your knowledge and make reasonable checks to make sure any information you give is accurate.

Figure 4.5 Excerpt from Domain 4: Maintaining Trust.

Source: (GMP 2013, p. 21) Copyright General Medical Council, reproduced with permission.

adopted this style of writing, which has served to imply the existence of a contract between individuals (i.e. students, employees) and the respective institution to which they belong. This reflects the insidious atmosphere of litigation that, I argue, is increasingly encroaching on our lives and relationships and which has come to define the way in which we engage with each other in the wider world. The public failings of healthcare systems, as identified through numerous public inquiries – Bristol heart inquiry (DOH 2001), Rodney Ledward (DOH 2000), Harold Shipman (Smith 2002), Mid Staffordshire NHS Trust (Francis 2013) – have played a significant role in creating a culture of legalification, which is meant to ensure accountability in practice.

A physician has to demonstrate compliance with *all GMP* criteria to be allowed to continue to practice. This is the foundation for appraisal and revalidation. Whilst the intentions behind *GMP* (2013) are worthy, notably to remove doubt regarding the expectations of minimum standards in practice, the highly didactic content and prescriptive format fails to capture the complexity of actual events of clinical practice and, as such, the document may be providing inadequate preparation for the reality of medical practice.

4.4   Care constituted as a cultural process

There is a wide body of literature on clinical communication skills and how to facilitate constructive doctor-patient interaction (Lloyd et al 2018; Brown and Bylund 2008). Doctors can have excellent communication skills and demonstrate optimal body language, which, though desirable, is not an end in itself. Possession of these skills does not necessarily translate into success when giving care. I was proud of the rapport I had established with Mr. Pitt and the clarity and compassion of my communications with him; however it did not ensure a successful outcome. The GMC patient feedback questionnaire (see Figure 4.6) identifies what the regulator views as important or necessary when assessing how a doctor engages in a patient consultation. It begins by posing questions regarding the personal conduct of the doctor and ends with how the doctor performed as a whole. This document defines conduct through three criteria: are they courteous ('polite'), attentive ('did they listen') and comforting ('make you feel at ease').

I have worked as a surgeon on two other continents, South Asia (Sri Lanka) and North America (New York), where the aforementioned 'niceties' would not be considered important or integral to framing good clinical interaction. In the UK, these qualities are rooted in a historical tradition of pleasantry unique to the British 'way of life' and, as such, have cultural significance and value. The inclusion of these qualities in the questionnaire provide an understanding of how care is socially constructed within British society. The authors of the questionnaire may argue that the manifestation of these qualities by a physician indicate respect for the patient and pre-empt good communication. I do not doubt this. But it is important to understand that the incorporation of these qualities in the document suggests how the regulators and therefore the official body of medicine identifies the *visible face* of 'care': socially constituted by cultural virtues.

4	How good was your doctor today at each of the following? (Please tick one box in each line)						
		Poor	Less than satisfactory	Satisfactory	Good	Very good	Does not apply
a	Being polite	☐	☐	☐	☐	☐	☐
b	Making you feel at ease	☐	☐	☐	☐	☐	☐
c	Listening to you	☐	☐	☐	☐	☐	☐
d	Assessing your medical condition	☐	☐	☐	☐	☐	☐
e	Explaining your condition and treatment	☐	☐	☐	☐	☐	☐
f	Involving you in decisions about your treatment	☐	☐	☐	☐	☐	☐
g	Providing or arranging treatment for you	☐	☐	☐	☐	☐	☐

Figure 4.6 GMC Patient Feedback Questionnaire (2014).

Source: Copyright General Medical Council, reproduced with permission.

I know from my own experience of being a patient that polite and attentive clinicians can still leave me feeling empty and disconnected from the substance of the encounter. Therefore, in order to understand how a patient experiences care, one must appreciate the need for professional codes of behaviour whilst also being sensitive to cultural prerequisites and external rules of conduct imposed by regulatory bodies. This allows for discovery of what is important to the individual patient and how that consultation *matters* to him. Yet again, how something matters to an individual cannot be foreseen nor predicted and resists attempts to be adequately captured by a series of guidelines.

4.5   *Good Surgical Practice (GSP)* (2014)

In September 2014, a number of surgical organisations[2] collaborated to write and produce *Good Surgical Practice* (2014), which I abbreviate to *GSP*. The document sought to make the guidance and standards outlined in *GMP* relevant to surgeons engaged in surgical practice. *GSP* opens with the following statement:

We share the privilege of working as surgeons, with the responsibilities, joys and disappointments that this brings. As surgeons we understand the fulfilment of delivering a successful outcome, and the humility and strength required when surgery goes wrong or is unlikely to be a patient's best option. We are all human, we all make mistakes and so we all benefit from guidance. We are fortunate; our profession is still respected and held in high esteem. Our behaviours and attitudes are observed by those we work alongside and impact directly on the care we deliver to our patients. The challenge of providing compassionate, high quality, safe care is at the top of our professional agenda.

(ibid., 4)

It conveys a romanticised notion of the surgeon as noble, embattled, good but fallible. It clothes the profession in virtuous robes: 'strength', 'humility', 'respect' and 'compassion'. The symbolic evocation of the virtuous yet fallible surgeon may appeal to the emotional core of the profession's members. Through this statement, the RCS communicates to all surgeons through a personal voice that acknowledges the challenges and complexities of their everyday practice. It reinforces a sense that surgeons are united (constant repetition of 'we') by their common *affective* experiences of surgical practice; that is, it conveys how the demands and the joys of a career in surgery make them *feel*. I use the terms 'feel' or 'feelings' in accordance with a definition provided by Whitehead (1929) in his theory of experience, that is, the way in which one encounters something (object or event) and how it comes to matter to that individual (e.g. the pleasure felt when one encounters a beautiful flower). The 'pleasure' is sensed and perceived by the body even before one is cognisant of 'beauty' as a concept. Put another way, an individual experiences the beauty of the flower before cognitive factors intervene to describe and organise that experience.

By creating an affective connection with its readership, *GSP* signals how it can be relevant to surgeons from all disciplines; it claims to understand what is at the heart of surgical practice.

It goes on to state the objectives:

> *Good Surgical Practice* aims to be a base line of clear and assessable standards for individual surgeons and their practice. It is not a statutory code or a regulatory document but rather seeks to exemplify the standards required of all doctors by the GMC in the context of surgery. It represents the profession's core values, the skills and attitudes that underpin surgical professionalism to which all surgeons should aspire in order to deliver high quality care.
>
> (p. 4)

The authors claim that, while the document is not a regulatory text, it outlines the minimum standard of practice expected of surgeons by the RCS and the GMC. By claiming to represent the 'profession's core values', the RCS appoints itself as the official voice of the profession, that is, the authority on what is deemed by surgeons to be important, what skills and attitudes they must demonstrate in practice and what ethical principles shape their everyday practice.[3] I explore how the notion of an ethics of practice had been captured by the RCS through this written guidance and what a surgeon might infer from it. The next subsection critiques how the text interprets and conceptualises an ethics of practice and why its approach is problematic.

The 'profession's core values'

The launch of this document was accompanied by a three-and-a-half-minute promotional video.[4] A senior medical director at the University Hospital of South Manchester makes the following comment:

> The NHS for a long time has accepted poor values and standards and individual surgeons have produced huge amount of variation in practise, a variation in standards which has led to a variation in outcomes and the Royal College's Standards (team) have produced a framework of values really. Its values as much as rules I think, which will enable surgeons to practise so much more safely in the future.

Clare Marx, the then president of the RCS is filmed, stating that

> We can no longer allow people to vacillate about whether this is important or not important. The general view is, a bit like washing your hands, this is something you just have to do . . . it's not actually just about checking, it's about the whole ethos of the safety culture, it's about the whole business of team working, it's about the whole open to challenge and it's about learning from other people and making sure that the patient lies at the heart of it and that that patient is safe.

These comments describe the tolerance of poor practices, acceptance of low expectations and reliance on the approaches of individual surgeons (i.e. as opposed to a unified professional stance on what is deemed acceptable practice and what is not), which reflect the findings of the Mid Staffordshire inquiry (Francis 2013). The subsequent responses from the college and government saw the romanticised service of surgeons, which was iterated in the opening pages, replaced with the more prosaic categories of the GMC regulations: 'standards', 'framework of values', 'rules', 'business', 'team working' and 'safety.' The text has created two worlds of surgery. The first is romantic and idealised, while the second is flawed and in need of urgent repair. The repair, at the suggestion of the RCS, comes in the form of guidance provided by *GSP*.

Through an external framework of standards, rules, regulations and a non-negotiable code of conduct (e.g. 'we can no longer allow people to vacillate'), the RCS, through *GSP*, attempts to remedy what is wrong with modern surgical practice. The text presents a code of conduct similar to *GMP* and one that is exhaustive, listing every detail of the practical aspects of a surgeon's day-to-day routine. For example, in Domain 1 (knowledge, skills, competence), it instructs surgeons to write clearly and legibly when listing the appropriate date and patient details:

1.3 Record your work clearly, accurately and legibly

Ensure that all medical records are accurate, clear, legible, comprehensive and contemporaneous and have the patient's identification details on them.

Ensure that a record is made by a member of the surgical team of important events and communications with the patient or supporter (for example, prognosis or potential complication). Any change in the treatment plan should be recorded.

(GSP 2014, p. 21)

I suggest that the challenge confronting this document, similar to *GMP*, is finding ways to accommodate the principles of practice and the inviolate ethics of conduct without diluting this message via the inclusion of operational details of day-to-day working, also presented as core values to abide by. By providing rigid rules and specifics on how surgeons must conduct themselves, it fails to distinguish between 'a principle' and 'a technique'. Autonomous individuals like surgeons, who deal with complex practice every day and must, in accordance, use independent judgment, do require overarching principles that can guide, inform and assist their practice. They should also be free to use whatever technique is appropriate given the circumstances to achieve those principles. For example, rather than outlining the specific techniques a surgeon should use to achieve the goal of clear communication, I would instead identify the overarching principle of 'ensure[ing] communications are clear and understood' to illustrate a key value. By contrast, the excerpt from *GSP* is an operational technique. Cultivating appropriate and compassionate professional values requires understanding that guidelines in addition to being instructive must also be aspirational and inspirational. This mean acknowledging that professional guidance must support practice but also encourage creativity to innovate and extend what providing care can mean in the modern age.

In the next chapter I explore how these guidelines are enacted in real examples of practice. I pose the following questions: how do the rules and recommendations translate when immersed in complex clinical encounters where it is not always clear how to proceed? Are there other factors that impact how a clinician chooses to act? Are these influences accommodated or recognised by the official handbooks of practice?

Notes

1   A detailed discussion on what constitutes professional misconduct is beyond the scope of this book. However, the expression 'serious professional misconduct' was substituted by the Medical Act of 1969 for the term 'infamous conduct in a professional respect', used in the Medical Act of 1858. It infers an act of omission, negligence or incompetence which falls below the standards set by the governing body, the GMC (Hamer 2010).

2   The Association of Surgeons of Great Britain and Ireland
The British Association of Oral and Maxillofacial Surgeons
The British Association of Otorhinolaryngologists – Head and Neck Surgeons

The British Association of Paediatric Surgeons
The British Association of Plastic, Reconstructive and Aesthetic Surgeons
The British Association of Urological Surgeons
The British Orthopaedic Association
The Royal College of Physicians and Surgeons of Glasgow
The Royal College of Surgeons in Ireland
The Royal College of Surgeons of Edinburgh
The Society for Cardiothoracic Surgery in Great Britain and Ireland
The Society of British Neurological Surgeons
The Vascular Society of Great Britain and Ireland

3   As explained previously, the RCS is the professional body responsible for surgical exams, awarding higher surgical qualifications and setting the content of the surgical curriculum. The primary responsibility of the RCS is to patients and the improvement of patient care, for which it was given a royal charter. Its engagement with surgeons is through ways that will ultimately affect the care of patients, such as running courses and trainings to develop and consolidate surgical skills, thus improving clinical outcomes and patient experience.

4   www.rcseng.ac.uk/surgeons/surgical-standards/professionalism-surgery/gsp/gsp

References

Bradley, E. H., Cherlin, E., McCorkle, R., Fried, T. R., Kasl, S. V., Cicchetti, D. V., et al. (2001). "Nurses' Use of Palliative Care Practices in the Acute Care Setting. *Journal of Professional Nursing*, 17: 14–22.

Brown, R. F., and Bylund, C. L. (2008). "Communication Skills Training: Describing a New Conceptual Model." *Academic Medicine*, 83 (10): 37–44.

Cleland, J., Reeve, J., et al. (2014). "Resisting the Tick Box Culture: Refocusing Medical Education and Training." *British Journal of General Practice*, 64 (625): 422–423.

Corrado, M. (2011). "No-One Likes Us, or Do They?" *Science and Public Affairs*, August: 14–15.

Cribb, A., and Entwistle, V. A. (2011). "Shared Decision-Making: Trade-Offs Between Narrower and Broader Conceptions." *Health Expectations*, 14: 210–219.

Department of Health. (2000). *The Report of the Inquiry into Quality and Practice Within the National Health Service Arising from the Actions of Rodney Ledward* (The Ritchie report). London: Stationery Office.

Department of Health. (2001). *Report of the Public Inquiry into Children's Heart Surgery at the Bristol Royal Infirmary 1984–1995: Learning from Bristol* (The Kennedy report). London: Stationery Office.

Dworkin, G. (1992). "Paternalism." In Becker, L. (Ed.), *Encyclopaedia of Ethics* (pp. 939–942). New York: Garland Publishing.

Epstein, R. M., and Street, R. L. (2011). "The Values and Value of Patient-Centered Care." *Annals of Family Medicine*, 9: 100–103.

Faubion, J. D. (Ed.). (2002). *Michel Foucault Power: Essential Works of Foucault 1954–1984, Vol. 3*. New York: Penguin Books.

Flin, R., Youngson, G., and Yule, S. (2007). "How Do Surgeons Make Intraoperative Decisions?" *Quality & Safety Health Care*, 16: 235–239.

Francis, Sir Robert. (2013). *The Report of the Mid Staffordshire NHS Foundation Trust Public Inquiry. Executive Summary*. London: The Stationary Office.

Frank, C., Asp, M., and Dahlberg, K. (2009). "Patient Participation in Emergency Care – A Phenomenographic Analysis of Caregivers' Conceptions." *Journal of Clinical Nursing*, 18: 2555–2562.

General Medical Council. (1993). *Tomorrow's Doctors: Recommendations on Undergraduate Medical Education*. London: General Medical Council.

General Medical Council. (1995). *Good Medical Practice*. London: General Medical Council.

General Medical Council. (1998). *Good Medical Practice*. London: General Medical Council.

General Medical Council. (2001). *Good Medical Practice*. London: General Medical Council.

General Medical Council. (2006). *Good Medical Practice*. London: General Medical Council.

General Medical Council. (2010). *To Consider the Review of Good Medical Practice*, 27 October. London: General Medical Council.

General Medical Council. (2013). *Good Medical Practice*. General Medical Council.

General Medical Council. (2016). *Promoting Excellence: Standards for Medical Education and Training*. Retrieved from www.gmc-uk.org/Promoting_excellence_standards_for_medical_education_and_training_0715.pdf_61939165.pdf.

Guenter, D., Fowler, N., and Lee, L. (2011). "Clinical Uncertainty: Helping Our Learners." *Canadian Family Physician*, 57 (1): 120–122.

Health Foundation. (2016). *Introduction to Person-Centred Care*. Retrieved from http://personcentredcareintro.health.org.uk.

Jalote-Parmar, A., and Badke-Schaub, P. (2008). *Critical Factors Influencing Intra-Operative Surgical Decision-Making*. International Conference on Systems, Man and Cybernetics, Singapore, 12–15 October, pp. 1091–1096.

Judge, K., and Solomon, M. (1993). "Public Opinion and the National Health Service: Patterns and Perspectives in Consumer Satisfaction." *Journal of Social Policy*, 22 (3): 299–327.

Jung, H. P., Wensing, M., and Grol, R. (1998). "What Makes a Good General Practitioner: Do Patients and Doctors Have Different Views?" *British Journal of General Practice*, 47: 805–809.

Kitson, A. (2016). "Why Do We Need to Study the Fundamentals of Care?" *Canadian Journal of Nursing Leadership*, 29: 10–16.

Kitson, A., Conroy, T., Wengstrom, Y., Profetto-McGrath, J., and Robertson-Malt, S. (2010). "Defining the Fundamentals of Care." *International Journal of Nursing Practice*, 16, 423–434.

Kret, D. D. (2011). "The Qualities of a Compassionate Nurse According to the Perceptions of Medical-Surgical Patients." *Medical-Surgical Nursing*, 20 (1): 29–36.

Latifi, R., Greussner, R., and Rhee, P. (2013). "Intraoperative Decision-Making Process: The Art and the Science." In Latifi, R. (Eds.), *Surgery for Complex Abdominal Wall Defects* (pp. 1–4). New York: Springer.

Leininger, M. (2001). *Culture Care Diversity and Universality: A Theory of Nursing*. New York: National League for Nursing Press.

Lloyd, M., Bor, R., and Noble, L. (2018). *Clinical Communication Skills for Medicine* (4th ed.). Elsevier.

Logan, R. L., and Scott, P. J. (1996). "Uncertainty in Clinical Practice: Implications for Quality and Costs of Health Care." *Lancet*, 347 (9001): 595–598.

McKinstry, B. (1992). "Paternalism and the Doctor-Patient Relationship in General Practice." *British Journal of General Practice*, 42 (361): 340–342.

O'Neill, O. (1984). "Paternalism and Partial Autonomy." *Journal of Medical Ethics*, 10: 173–178.

Papadopoulos, I., Taylor, G., Ali, S., et al. (2015). "Exploring Nurses' Meaning and Experiences of Compassion: An International Online Survey Involving 15 Countries." *Journal of Transcultural Nursing*, 28 (3): 286–295.

Pauley, K., Flin., R., et al. (2011). "Surgeons' Intraoperative Decision Making and Risk Management." *American Journal of Surgery*, 202: 375–381.

Picker Europe. (2006). *Engaging Patients in Their Healthcare: How Is the UK Doing Relative to Other Countries*. Retrieved from www.pickereurope.org/wp-content/uploads/2014/10/Engaging-patients-in-their-healthcare-how-is-the-UK-doing . . . . pdf.

Roach, M. S. (1997). *Caring from the Heart: The Convergence of Caring and Spirituality*. New York: Paulist Press.

Royal College of Surgeons of England. (2014). *Good Surgical Practice*. RCSE: Professional Standards.

Siegler, M. (1985). "The Progression of Medicine: From Physician Paternalism to Patient Autonomy to Bureaucratic Parsimony." *Archives of Internal Medicine*, 145 (4): 713–715.

Smith, J. (2002). *The Shipman Inquiry. First Report. Volume One. Death Disguised*. Manchester: The Shipman Inquiry.

Stronach, I. (2010). *Globalising Education, Educating the Local: How Method Made Us Mad*. Routledge.

Sutton, P. A., Hornby, S. T., et al. (2015). "Instinct, Intuition and Surgical Decision-Making." *Royal College of Surgeons Bulletin*, 97 (8): 345–347.

van der Cingel, M. (2011). "Compassion in Care: A Qualitative Study of Older People with a Chronic Disease and Nurses." *Nursing Ethics*, 18 (5): 672–685.

Watson, J. (2008). *Nursing: The Philosophy and Science of Caring* (rev. ed.). Boulder: University Press of Colorado.

West, A. F., and West, R. R. (2002). "Clinical Decision-Making: Coping with Uncertainty." *Postgraduate Medical Journal*, 78: 319–321.

Whitehead, A. N. (1929). *Process and Reality*. New York: The Free Press.

Wolf, A., Moore, L., et al. (2017). "The Realities of Partnership in Person-Centred Care: A Qualitative Interview Study with Patients and Professionals." *British Medical Journal Open*, 7: e016491. doi:10.1136/bmjopen-2017-016491.

5 Negotiating and Coping with Complex Events of Practice and Difficult Conversations

The 'Errant' Testicle

We were both scrutinizing the operating field. In this case it comprised a 35-year-old man's lower abdomen, or groin (as commonly termed), and the contents of his spermatic cord (a rope-like structure that proceeds from the tissues of the lower abdomen to the testicles in the scrotum and carries the vas deferens, that is, a white tube that carries sperm). The scheduled operation was 'surgical repair of an inguinal, or, groin hernia'. A hernia occurs due to a weakness in the abdominal wall, leading to the contents of the abdomen (such as bowel or fat) pushing through into the tissues of the groin. This typically presents as a protruding lump that is more prominent when standing, straining or coughing. However, 15 minutes into the operation, we were both stumped. We had identified the weakness in the wall and were trying to identify what exactly was herniating into the groin. What we found was a rather small, shrivelled, egg-like structure ensconced in the spermatic cord.

"That's a testicle!" we both chimed. "My goodness, how long has that been there for?!" Answer: since he left the womb.

During pregnancy, a male foetus' testicles travel from a site within the abdomen to the scrotum. There is sometimes a delay of this process, so that at birth the testicles have not yet descended (travelled to the scrotum). However, after six months of age, if a single or pair of testicles have not yet descended, the standard practice is to identify where they are sitting (usually still in the lower abdomen), bring one or both into the scrotal sac and stitch both into their proper place within the scrotum. Why? The established research demonstrates that after six months of age, undescended testes rarely descend spontaneously into the scrotum. They remain in the abdomen, where they can be a cause for reduced fertility and, more importantly, put the individual at high risk of testicular cancer. For these reasons male infants with a missing testicle(s) are investigated and, if necessary, a surgery will follow.

"I didn't examine his scrotum. I should have, but it seemed quite full," MB (consultant) admitted, sadly. Scrotal examination is part of the physical examination of a patient with a hernia, but it is often missed if there appears to be no need, especially as the examination of intimate areas can create anxiety and embarrassment for the patient. At this point, I pulled down the drapes and examined his scrotum. There was indeed just one unusually large testicle present.

"Well the scrotum appears deceptively normal because the one testicle he does have is so big!" I conceded. "It changes nothing, however. We still have to remove this testicle, because it's a risk for cancer and, besides, it's been non-functional for the past 35 years. It is unexpected, but we've done this young man some good today," I concluded.

The rest of the operation proceeded fairly uneventfully. It wasn't until later, when we were both completing the paperwork for the surgery, that I found myself, for the second time that day, completely astonished. While filling in the theatre record on the computer, I casually asked MB, "so what will you tell him (the patient)?" He looked up at me nonchalantly while composing the operative note on paper, rubbed his eyes and said very matter of factly, "oh nothing, it's not relevant, we did him no harm today . . . in fact we protected him by doing this operation . . . he was at risk of a cancer, but not anymore . . . he doesn't need to know, it will only upset him and make him uncomfortable. We've treated his problem." With that final word, he returned to his writing.

I was gobsmacked.

"But doesn't he have a right to know? I'm sure we won't alarm him if we tell him that the lump was caused by a missing testicle . . . in fact he may tell us that he always wondered why he had just one ball?! We can tell him that we did him some good today." Even as I spoke these words, I knew from his body language that such a conversation was not to happen. Ever. I continued to watch him. Under 'Procedure name,' he wrote slowly and purposefully, 'Orchiectomy (removal of testis) and repair of inguinal hernia.' He murmured without looking up from his writing, "I don't think that's necessary." That was that.

This narrative from my surgical journal is an example of how a surgeon responds when confronted by the thisness of an unexpected event within a clinical encounter. In coping with an unfamiliar situation, how the surgeon experiences the event and engages with the encounter (*affective* relations) may trigger ways of responding (i.e. thinking, acting) that she had not conceived of prior to the event. Earlier in the chapter I discussed how authorised manuals of practice (Official Care) do not fully capture the complexity of actual events of practice (Real Care). I now investigate the response to an encounter of Real Care (providing care in contingent events) in relation to the recommendations of Official Care, that being what is set out in clinical guidelines and ethical codes.

The unexpected event was the discovery of a testicle in an otherwise routine hernia surgery. MD, the senior surgeon, is an inspiring and compelling figure. No patient leaves his clinic without a diagnosis or a clear plan to establish a diagnosis. He is careful to elicit important details when a patient describes his health problems. He is compassionate to distressed patients, sensitive to the impact of their condition and zealous in the pursuit of treatment and cure. Therefore, why did he not inform the patient of the discovery (i.e. a non-functioning testicle in a hernia sac)? Is it because, as he stated, it was 'not relevant'? Certainly, removing a non-functional testicle that the patient was unaware of, and which contributed nothing to his health, had no adverse outcome. In fact, by removing the testicle, MD had eliminated the risk of it becoming cancerous in the future. Perhaps, these issues motivated his belief that the operative finding was 'irrelevant'. But the crucial question in this and every clinical encounter between doctor and patient is whether the surgeon's course of action was ethically sound. Did MD fulfil his ethical duty to the patient? What conduct constitutes the ethical act of the surgeon?

5.1 Candid conversations

> You must be honest and trustworthy in all your communication with patients and colleagues.
>
> (GMC 2013, p. 21)

Over almost three decades public inquiries into adverse events or appalling standards of care have placed an intense scrutiny on healthcare practices. Most recently the Mid Staffordshire inquiry, led by Sir Francis (2013), identified serious failings in health and social care at the NHS trust. These failings led to unacceptable patient harm resulting in 'appalling suffering' as well as patient deaths. This inquiry, in addition to many other incidents over the course of a decade, placed a spotlight on harmful practices in healthcare. The Francis report (2013) attributed the failures partly to a working culture that lacked openness, transparency and honesty in practice. This culture, the report suggested, created a decaying environment that was fertile for wilful neglect, poor practice, mistakes and errors. Government policy and further inquiries explored measures to combat dangerous attitudes and practices in healthcare (DOH 2014a, 2014b). An example of the resulting proposals is the overall objective to create 'a culture of candour' in clinical environments (DOH 2014a, 2014b, 2014c; RCS 2015), one that would make unsafe and potentially harmful situations unacceptable. The overall outcome was the widespread initiative to place 'patient safety' at the centre of all systems, practices and training.

In late 2014, this culminated in new legislation through the introduction of a *statutory Duty of Candour* for all healthcare professionals and organisations involved in patient care (House of Commons 2014, p. 24):

1 [Registered persons] must act in an open and transparent way with relevant persons in relation to care and treatment provided to service users in carrying on a regulated activity.

The *Duty of Candour* (2015) document published by the RCS is primarily concerned with promoting honest communications when serious errors or adversity have occurred: 'a *notifiable safety incident*, i.e. an incident that resulted or has the potential to result in moderate harm, severe harm or death' (ibid., 9, my emphasis). However, the document does state that, 'after the surgical procedure, the surgeon has a duty towards his or her patient to give an account of what happened during the operation' (RCS 2015, p. 8).

MD did meet with the patient afterwards in the recovery area and gave him a brief and reassuring account of the surgery. Critically, he did not divulge the surprising finding of an errant testicle. It could be assumed that a description of what occurred in a clinical procedure or treatment, or during the sequence of events that led to a particular outcome (good or bad), should be a simple matter of speaking the *truth* (i.e. that which happened). The fact that this did not happen raises the question of *whose interests were served* by an omission of the full facts in this case? To answer this I offer an alternative theory, one based upon the fact that MD appeared to believe that full disclosure of the procedure would have caused the patient unnecessary distress and confusion.

Difficult conversations

Perhaps the surgeon, MD, imagined the following conversation:

Surgeon: A funny thing . . . we found a testicle in your hernia.

Patient: My testicle? What do you mean? You took my testicle out?!!

Surgeon: Yes, but also, no. We found that you had one testicle in your scrotum and the second one was hiding inside your belly.

Patient: But I don't understand, I've always had two testicles. Why did you take the second one out? Now I've only got one testicle. I thought you were operating on my hernia?

Surgeon: No, you've only got one testicle. The second one had not fully descended into your scrotum when you were a child. But don't worry, you'll be just fine. You know it's a good thing we took it out, because it could have become a cancer.

Patient: Cancer? You mean I might have cancer? But I came in today because you told me I had a hernia!

There are many conversations in routine practice that resemble this: complex, complicated and ripe for miscommunication and misunderstanding. It is well established and extensively covered in the literature that communicating either complicated information or bad news is an area of difficulty, distress and reluctance for most clinicians (Maguire et al. 1986; Dosanjh et al. 2001; Fallowfield and Jenkins 2004; Barnett et al. 2007; Turini et al. 2008; Herbert et al. 2009). Physicians are faced with the dual challenge of managing the turmoil of a patient's emotions (e.g. shock, anger, grief) as well as coping with personal feelings of disappointment, guilt and sadness.

Rigorous training in communication skills and the development of practical algorithms help prepare physicians and also simplify potentially difficult conversations or clinical events into framed structures. However, these measures cannot accurately account for either the intricacies of human expectation and understanding or how an event actually transpires. The nature of complex interactions is that they cannot be reduced to discrete categories, nor can their outcome be pre-judged.

Candour

I certainly believe that the established guidance is clear for this particular scenario as to what the standard of practice should be: MD must communicate the operative finding to the patient, thereby demonstrating transparency in his practice. It is possible that MD did not consider the encounter with an unexpected operative finding an adverse event and therefore felt it did not qualify for such a conversation. However, I strongly believe that efforts to further explicate or elucidate terms such as 'adversity', 'harm' or even 'candour', as advocated by some consultation documents (Dalton and Williams 2014), will not necessarily create more clarity for the physician, nor will it provide inducements to engage honestly and openly with patients.

This is not to discount existing measures established to identify and remove those attitudes and behaviours that foster and legitimise intolerable standards of care. Instead, I argue that an approach that single-mindedly pursues the development and enforcement of yet more clinical guidance and highly specified criteria is indifferent to the reality of medical encounters. This approach neglects to understand how the complexities of actual practice *affect* the ways in which professionals respond and react in difficult and challenging situations of Real Care. To illustrate this I outline some of the factors possibly implicated in MD's actions, using Giles Deleuze's theory of ethics (Smith 2007; Deleuze 1994).

5.2   An ethics of immanence

The earlier discussion identifies two ideologies of ethical practice. In the first, ethics is defined as an uncompromising code of conduct that is grounded in Kantian principles of morality. A physician's actions are assessed according to moral criteria, which evaluate and judge the intentions, thoughts and behaviours along categories of 'right' and 'wrong'. Deleuze (Smith 2007) opines that ethics based on morality reflect the transcendent framework of values held by society at that moment in time. Deleuze uses the term 'transcendent', here, to describe the approved system of morals established within society. This structure of values is expected to direct and influence how individuals and organisations think and 'do'.

The second ideology of ethics emerges from real events of clinical practice, in which a doctor is forced to make decisions in the 'here and now', or, haecceities of an encounter, according to the contingencies of the actual doctor-patient relationship. To explore Deleuze's notion of ethics, I draw upon the writings of Daniel Smith, who provides excellent insights into some of Deleuze's denser theory.

> What he (Deleuze) calls 'ethics', is on the contrary, a set of 'facilitative' [*facultative*] rules that evaluates what we do, say, and think according to the

immanent mode of existence that it implies. One says or does this, thinks or feels that: what mode of existence does it imply? 'We always have the beliefs, feelings, and thoughts we deserve', writes Deleuze, 'given our way of being or our style of life'.

(Smith 2007, p. 67)

An 'immanent mode of existence' is at the heart of Deleuze's conception of ethics, but what does this actually mean? Notions of ethics, for Deleuze, are intimately linked to an individual's *capacity to act* and the *affective relations* that enable or diminish the *power* to act.

To return to the narrative example, to understand the actions of MD is to explore how he *prehends* (Whitehead 1929) an event. 'Prehension' is a term introduced by Alfred Whitehead to denote how one entity *takes account of* another entity (see Chapters 2 and 3). For example, performing an operation involves a sequence of prehensive relations involving the organic and non-organic components that constitute the act of operating. Put simply, there are intricate networks of relations involving the rotational action of the wrist, the scalpel, sutures, blood, tissue, memories of previous procedures, frustrations and surprises, for example. These entities intermingle and also pull apart and act on each other in complex tiers of *intra-action* (Barad 2007). Such a process characterises the act and experience of operating. It is difficult to know precisely how these relations influence an individual to think or act in a specific way. However, I suggest that these relations are involved in how an individual engages with an event, because they constitute how something comes to matter to her.

In the narrative of the hernia operation, how does MD prehend the surgical encounter? What affects him in the encounter? Is he affected by the surprising discovery of the testicle? What affects diminish or augment his capacity to act in this example of practice? These questions emphasise the *affective conditions* that constitute his capacity to act and how he engages with the encounter: 'we arrive at a real definition of a mode of existence only when we define it in terms of its power or capacity to be affected [. . .] what is it affected by in the world? What leaves it unaffected?' (Smith 2012, p. 154). The power to act in a given moment is not determined by 'logical possibility' (i.e. what we are told, know or conceive to be possible); rather it is sparked by what the person is actually *enabled* to think and do, and how they are *enabled* to react or respond at every moment (what is actualised).

Thus, an ethics of immanence refers to the capacity to be affected in ways that encourage an individual to ask in a given moment or situation, *'what can I do, what am I capable of doing?'* (Smith 2007, p. 67, my emphasis). Critics have accused Deleuze and Foucault of peddling 'immorality' by introducing a philosophy that rejects normative criteria used to judge thoughts or actions. It is beyond the scope of this book to look carefully at all of Deleuze's arguments; however, one of his rebuttals to the aforementioned criticism is significant to the narrative presented herein, and therefore I develop this here.

A particular mode of existence can, indeed, be assessed along established moral criteria (transcendent frameworks) that judge intentions and actions as 'good' or 'bad' depending on how closely they comply with the external system of approved values. But an ethics of immanence is distinguished by the *singularity of an event* – the specific situation that an individual finds himself in at a given moment. Put another way, 'the object of philosophy is not to contemplate the eternal, nor to reflect on history, but to diagnose our actual becomings' (Deleuze and Guattari 1994).

An ethics of immanence requires a physician at every moment to ask, 'What is in my power to do such that I reach the limits of my capabilities?'. What I advocate in this book is an approach that encourages physicians to ask, 'In this event of practice, have I pushed myself to do all that I can?'

'Doing the right thing' is defined via a moral stance that is premised on known and approved outcomes that pre-exist an event. It is founded on a framework of predefined values to establish acceptable and safe practices. However, broad application of a universal system of pre-approved, transcendent values can potentially limit the intrinsic and actual capacities of an individual in two ways. First, a rigid classification of 'good' and 'bad' practice may dissuade a physician from being *responsive* or from effectively engaging with an encounter. This is because the physician's 'natural' inclination or response in a situation is not recognised or accommodated by the authorised forms of conduct. Second, responding in a manner that transcends established protocols is critical if new ways of being, thinking and doing are to suffuse medical practice and thereby enhance patient care and professional conduct.

5.3   The immanence of practice: 'Discognition'

In summary, each clinical encounter is charged with affective relations that can spark numerous ways of coping, acting and thinking at every moment. Steven Shaviro (2015) argues that, as *sentient beings*, our initial experiencing of the world is not necessarily conscious, rational or immersed in cognitive thought. He contends that how we first come to know, understand and make sense of the world is grounded in aspects of sentience. These aspects include sensory awareness or arousal, which inform mental functioning and subjective experience.

Shaviro introduces the notion of 'discognition' as what *'disrupts cognition, exceeds the limits of cognition, but also subtends cognition'* (ibid., 10–11, my emphasis). He appears to suggest that sentient modes of thinking are not only prior to cognition but also have the potential to interrupt rational processes, subsequently reconfiguring how we 'think' on matters. Put another way, a state of discognition is a parallel mode of thinking. Sentience is a mode of 'thinking' that has yet to be captured by cognition or emotion. However, a transcendent framework of ethics sets out specific ways of thinking and practicing that may appear unconnected to the haecceities of real practice.

I advocate an approach that is sensitive to an ethics of immanence. In events of practice that are unanticipated or unexpected, there is a need to consider carefully the immanent nature of clinical relations and practice by relaxing the grip of transcendent frameworks. Both narratives depict the potential for unanticipated events of practice to generate affective states that can precipitate a renegotiation of the doctor-patient relationship.

5.4   Concluding remarks

In the two chapters that constitute the second part of this book, I have attempted to explore, through the central concept of care, the difference between how to give appropriate care in unanticipated or unpredictable clinical situations and how care is treated as a major concept within medical and clinical guidelines. In the former, the surgeon has to make decisions in unfamiliar situations, trying to find a way forward. The affects that lead to the thoughts and actions of the surgeon relate to an ethics of immanence. In the latter, a transcendent ethics is promoted, the result of which is an established code that surgeons must adhere to. I do not argue that a formal code of ethics is unimportant. Guidelines that result from such are indeed important, but in unfamiliar situations they may not help an individual to cope with that which happens in those interactions between surgeon and patient wherein there is a real need to find an effective resolution.

Attempts in medical practice to establish a clear set of criteria, by which the work of practitioners can be evaluated (i.e. visibly measured), is a response to the past problems and failures of health care. Given this background, the drive to assess and measure is understandable; strong arguments can be made for it being a desirable component of modern healthcare processes. However, the desire for clarity through performative assessments and measurements can obscure the complexities of actual clinical practice, as demonstrated in the personal narratives in this chapter.

A focus on the 'complicated processes' of care and on the specific issues concerning delivery of care constitutes a particular preoccupation with the general business of healthcare. In order to cultivate professionals who can respond appropriately in a clinical encounter with the necessary dynamism, creativity and compassion, surgical and medical education and training must embrace a paradigm that goes beyond a narrow understanding of competence and skills acquisition. What is necessary is a relaxation and softening of approaches that mandate conduct and behaviour.

> If there is one lesson to be learnt, I suggest it is that people must always come before numbers. It is the individual experiences that lie behind statistics and benchmarks and action plans that really matter, and that is what must never be forgotten when policies are being made and implemented.
>
> (Robert Francis 2013, p. 4)

The challenge inherent in creating a professional guide to practice that embodies a profession's purpose, standards and ethics is to represent these aspirations as the core values and themes that inspire the design and delivery of innovative and compassionate patient care. The danger lies in reducing such an important endeavour into a tedious framework that organises the minutiae of clinical work.

The next section of this book, Part 3, demonstrates that, despite the best intentions, a didactic guide to practice is easily overlooked by practicing clinicians who regard it as both removed from the realities of their daily experiences of practice, and also unaligned with their expectations of themselves.

References

Barad, K. (2007). *Meeting the Universe Halfway: Quantum Physics and the Entanglement of Matter and Meaning.* Duke University Press.

Barnett, M. M., Fisher, J. D., et al. (2007). "Breaking Bad News: Consultants' Experience, Previous Education and Views on Educational Format and Timing." *Medical Education,* 41: 947–956.

Dalton, D., and Williams, N. (2014). *Building a Culture of Candour, a Review of the Threshold for the Duty of Candour and of the Incentives for Care Organisations to Be Candid.* Royal College of Surgeons of England.

Deleuze, G., and Guattari, F. (1994). *What Is Philosophy?* trans. Tomlinson, H., and Burchell, G. New York: Fordham University Press.

Department of Health. (2014a). *Hard Truths, the Journey to Putting Patients First: Volume One of the Government Response to the Mid Staffordshire NHS Foundation Trust Public Inquiry.* Retrieved from www.gov.uk/government/uploads/system/uploads/attachment_data/file/270368/34658_Cm_8777_Vol_1_accessible.pdf.

Department of Health. (2014b). *Introducing the Statutory Duty of Candour: A Consultation on Proposals to Introduce a New CQC Registration Regulation.* Retrieved from www.gov.uk/government/uploads/system/uploads/attachment_data/file/295773/Duty_of_Candour_Consultation.pdf.

Department of Health. (2014c). *Building A Culture of Candour: A Review of the Threshold for the Duty of Candour and of the Incentives for Care Organisations to Be Candid.* Retrieved from www.rcseng.ac.uk/government-relations-and-consultation/documents/CandourreviewFinal.pdf.

Dosanjh, S., Barnes, J., and Bhandari, M. (2001). "Barriers to Breaking Bad News Among Medical and Surgical Residents." *Medical Education,* 35: 197–205.

Fallowfield, L., and Jenkins, V. (2004). "Communicating Sad, Bad, and Difficult News in Medicine." *Lancet,* 363: 312–319.

Francis, Sir Robert. (2013). *The Report of the Mid Staffordshire NHS Foundation Trust Public Inquiry. Executive Summary.* London: The Stationary Office.

General Medical Council. (2013). *Good Medical Practice.* London: General Medical Council.

Herbert, H. D., Butera, J. N., et al. (2009). "Are We Training Our Fellows Adequately in Delivering Bad News to Patients? A Survey of Hematology/Oncology Program Directors." *Palliative Medical Journal,* 12: 1119–1124.

House of Commons. (2014). *Health and Social Care Act 2008 (Regulated Activities) Regulations 2014.* Retrieved from www.cqc.org.uk/sites/default/files/20150510_hsca_2008_regulated_activities_regs_2104_current.pdf.

Maguire, P., Fairborn, S., and Fletcher, C. (1986). "Consultation Skills of Young Doctors: II-Most Young Doctors Are Bad at Giving Information." *British Medical Journal* (Clinical Research Edition), 292: 1576–1578.

Royal College of Surgeons of England. (2015). *Duty of Candour: Guidance for Surgeons and Employers. RCS: Professional Standards.* Retrieved from www.rcseng.ac.uk/news/docs/1-duty-of-candour-web-final.pdf.

Shaviro, S. (2015). *Discognition*. London: Repeater Books.

Smith, D. W. (2007). "Deleuze and the Question of Desire: Toward an Immanent Theory of Ethics." *Parrhesia*, 2: 66–78. Retrieved from http://philpapers.org/archive/SMIDAT-5.pdf.

Smith, D. W. (2012). *Essays on Deleuze*. Edinburgh University Press.

Turini, B., Martins, N. D., et al. (2008). "Communication in Medical Education: Experience, Structuring and New Challenges in Medical Curricula." *Brazilian Journal of Medical Education*, 32: 264–270.

Whitehead, A. N. (1929). *Process and Reality*. New York: The Free Press.

Part III

The Affective Conditions of Pedagogy and Practice

6 Beyond Pedagogical Aims

The role of subjectivity and affect in shaping the reality of surgical training

The three chapters that comprise this third part of the book problematise the nature of pedagogic practices in clinical training, an endeavour which allows for the wider exploration of how the ideas and experiences expressed in clinical encounters matter to a surgeon. In its simplest form, the term pedagogy refers to the craft of teaching, that is, what a teacher does to bring about learning in others. It encompasses the thinking and practices that are used by educators to support and understand the process of discovery being undertaken by their learners. 'Pedagogy needs to be explored through the thinking and practice of those educators who look to accompany learners; care for and about them; and bring learning into life' (Smith n.d.).

In the ensuing chapters, surgical training practices are scrutinised from two perspectives. First, the treatment of learning and teaching within the framework of pedagogic materials is examined to identify how trainees and trainers are constructed within curricular and assessment discourses. Second, accounts of clinical experiences from trainees and trainers are analysed to illuminate how surgeon subjectivities emerge when engaging with the thisness, or, concrete reality, of actual clinical practice. The objective of this discussion is to think critically and constructively beyond the established pedagogy, that is, to illuminate how the *affective conditions* of practice affect how we experience professional practice, and also how we construct and encounter our sense of self in the clinical world. Affective responses tend to be non-visible and intangible, ignored and obscured by the transcendent framings of clinical practice. Therefore, their power to shape, influence and determine our emotions, thoughts and actions in practice are neither obvious, accommodated for, nor easily anticipated.

I suggest that consideration of how learners actually experience events of clinical training, beyond how they are characterised in training materials, can lead to an improved understanding of how clinicians learn and cope with the ontological and ethical complexities embedded in actual encounters of clinical practice. Such consideration may help develop a better understanding of how we comprehend ourselves and the intricacies of others. It may also highlight how the relative neglect of such consideration, traditionally, has led to consistent patterns in the ways in which policy and the structures of healthcare have influenced trainees, affectively.

6.1 Subjectivities

At the heart of this consideration is a concern about the nature of trainee (and trainer) subjectivities. At this point I want to briefly clarify what I mean by the term 'subjectivity'. It broadly refers to a sense of self, that is, the beliefs, attitudes, outlooks, subconscious tendencies, convictions and understandings that people hold, and which contribute to a sense of who they are (Hall 2004). I articulate a particular view of subjectivity in this book, which follows Michel Foucault (1972, 1982) and Judith Butler (1997), to explore how trainer and trainee identities are constituted through discourses and practices. This analytical approach is useful when attempting to understand how subjectivities form and develop – what factors and processes contribute to (i) how surgeons are conceived by external bodies (such as the RCS) and (ii) the ways in which surgeons as human beings and professionals think, act and reflect on practice.

6.2 Interview analysis

The analysis and discussion are framed around two interview accounts provided by Scarlett, a senior surgeon in training, and Amy, an educator at the Royal College of Surgeons. The narrative accounts illustrate the strong emotions and impassioned thoughts that arise from the individual experiences of professional training and education. Scarlett, an ST7 trainee from the South of England, is exasperated and disappointed by the current selection process into surgical training. Whilst Amy is frustrated by how the outcomes-driven agenda in surgical education stifles opportunities to widen the scope of training and education for surgeons. I have treated both narratives as discursive practices. This means that the accounts in and of themselves create the reality of the training practices for these individuals and are not an embodiment of objective truth or motive. This form of narrative analysis is consistent with the theories of discourse proposed by Foucault (1972) and Butler (2005).

> To describe a formulation qua statement does not consist in analysing the relations between the author and what he (sic) says (or wanted to say, or said without wanting to); but in determining what position can and must be occupied by any individual *if he is to be the subject of it.*
>
> (Foucault 1972, pp. 95–96)

Foucault draws attention to the conditions that make possible 'what can be said' about something and 'who can speak it'. This is a call to recognise and contemplate the relations of power that influence, control and determine the statements and speech of a person. These considerations are identified by Foucault (and Butler) as 'regimes of truth' (Foucault 1975, p. 30), or the conditions and frameworks that produce a reality for the speaker. Therefore, I approached the narrative analysis in this chapter with the following question: *what controls and regulates how a trainee becomes visible within the current system of surgical training?* Put another way, *what organisational forces and structures have created the reality of clinical training demonstrated within these narratives?*

In Chapter 7, the discussion is furthered by asking, *what kind of surgery training and education is being created?* Through an examination of training practices, I investigate how assessment criteria and a syllabus (i.e. established training materials) treat or 'pedagogise' learners and teachers. This is achieved through a critical analysis of certain surgical training materials: the intercollegiate surgical curriculum (ISC), work-based assessments (WBAs) and surgical trainer standards.

In the final chapter to this part of the book I ask how the ideas and experiences expressed in clinical encounters *matter* to a surgeon, namely, how the examples of reported clinical practice are significant for that learner. I am not overly concerned with proving the veracity of these statements nor the accuracy of the details. Instead, I suggest that learning can also occur as a function of *mattering*, specifically, how something that attains significance for a learner (and therefore 'matters') can create forms of knowing, including forms which may have been previously unknown to the individual. This is not to diminish the importance or effectiveness of known and established forms of surgical teaching and learning. Rather, I propose an alternate yet complementary approach to conventional forms of surgical learning and teaching, one which exceeds an application of these established medical pedagogies and ways of knowing.

I begin, then, with an examination of how the formal *structurisation* of medical practice – the enactment of health policy, the organisation and deployment of hospital departments and the employment of an 'outcomes agenda' on patient care and training – controls actualisations of practice.

6.3   Scarlett's story: finding the good ones

What people would say is that they compare the system now (based on assessments and criteria for competencies) and they would say, "well at least it's fair, at least it's not nepotistic like the old system." . . . But my feeling is, and as someone who was a junior trainee before we had any of these systems of assessment, as a house officer (F1 doctor), somebody wrote a little paragraph about me at the end of my job, and that was that. As a woman in Medicine, who didn't go to private school or didn't know anybody in Medicine, I actually had a huge amount of support from all the consultants I worked for. And that wasn't for any other reason other than they recognised that I was hard working, loyal and dedicated, as well as being good at the job. They really were vying for me and encouraged me, which made a huge difference. But when MMC[1] came in, that was the real final death knell of that sort of thing, where your boss would phone up their colleague to say, "make sure you shortlist this one because she's good."

. . . I had a whole bunch of consultants who were massively supportive, and they'd phone me and say, "have you been shortlisted?" And I would burst into tears and say, "no!" and they would be absolutely outraged on my behalf, and say "I don't understand, why is the new system not working?!"

> But the trouble is . . . [this new system] completely removes from the process of picking doctors the genuine support of other doctors. And I really think that you and, I, or anybody else whom you would consider a good doctor, would be consistently picked out by others as a good doctor. We all know who's good and who's not up to par, we all know it! But there's no way under the current system of just doing that . . . of saying, "I'll take these eight trainees but not those two (because they're no good!)" . . . It's the same with nurses isn't it? . . . You know which ones are the good ones . . . when someone says, "oh so-and-so is the nurse on the ward," then it's understood that, (those tasks) will never get done! There's an understanding of people. Human beings understand each other, that some are lazy, others are competent. We understand that about each other, that's thousands and millennia of evolution. Then we're coming to a system where we take all that out in order to make it fair. And I understand that it's a really difficult balance to strike.

At several points in the interview, Scarlett's irritation and bewilderment at the selection system for entry into surgical training boiled over. Her criticisms of the unfairness of the new training system arose from her personal experience of not being selected for further training. This contrasts with her personal certainty that she is conscientious and diligent, 'a good doctor', a phrase she repeats several times in the full interview and which is confirmed by her senior colleagues who have supported her entry into surgical training. In Chapter 4, the notion of the 'good doctor', as described and promoted by *Good Medical Practice* (2013), suggests a candidate who meets the mandated criteria set out in this practice handbook. However, what Scarlett is asserting through the notion of goodness is a more nuanced interpretation of duty and responsibility which emerges from an inherent ability to 'get the job done'. I explore this issue further, later in this chapter, but for now I return to her narrative. What struck me as noteworthy in our conversation was her burning sense of betrayal, which other interviewees also felt and expressed. If she had the backing of all these senior surgeons, who, by virtue of their position as consultants (and therefore 'top surgeons') delivered surgical training and conferred legitimacy on her candidature, then why had the new training system similarly not approved her? These contrasting experiences of the new training system – she is more than good enough to enter training but has not been selected by the surgery programme – have constituted *the reality* of the training system for both Scarlett and the community of surgeons she works with. Before proceeding with the narrative analysis, it seems sensible to briefly review how the current system of surgical training came into place.

6.4   Modernising Medical Careers (MMC): competency-based training

Since the 1990s in the UK, strong efforts have been made to modernise systems of postgraduate medical training and education. Previous to this, there was neither a clear structure nor rules on how one progressed through training, an environment which heralded the beginning of a major period of transition in surgical education. In 1992, Kenneth Calman, the then Chief Medical Officer, set up a working group for this purpose. The aim was to bring postgraduate training in line with the requirements of the European medical directives (DOH 1993). The report proposed a streamlined, specialist training programme with a defined curriculum and minimum training period. Successful completion of the postgraduate programme would result in formal qualification as a specialist in that particular field. This new training system was to be defined by clear educational objectives, training agreements and a move towards ensuring that trainees were competent, irrespective of how long they had spent in training (DOH 1995).

In 2005, a new postgraduate training programme, Modernising Medical Careers (MMC), was instituted for all disciplines of Medicine (DOH 2003). The system introduced new ways of training and assessing trainees in all disciplines of medicine. The house-officer-grade doctor (i.e. first-year post-qualification from medical school) was replaced with the foundation year doctor. The latter, having graduated from medical school, was now required to demonstrate safe practice over two years, prior to being fully licensed as a practicing physician.

Specialist training was highly structured and defined with objectives and outcomes that formed the introduction of a *competency-based* model of medical education. Competence-based training (CBT) refers to *outcomes-based education* and *assessment*, whereby a trainee is expected to *demonstrate* what they have learned:

> not only must doctors have the technical competence to treat a patient but they must also understand why they are doing it; they should adopt appropriate critical thinking to what they are doing; use appropriate decision-making strategies; and adopt appropriate attitudes to their patients.
>
> (Davis et al. 2007, p. 342)

Whilst, competency-based training (CBT) defines modern medical training, controversy continues as to its appropriateness as a model for medical education and its effectiveness in ensuring the aptitude and safety of trainees (Lurie 2011; Albanese et al. 2008; Touchie and Ten Cate 2016). In addition, to a further restructuring of training grades, MMC established a *certificate of completion of training* (CCT) awarded on successful completion of specialist surgical training. CCT is a mandatory requirement for any trainee expecting to assume consultant duties.

MMC was reviewed in an independent inquiry led by Professor Sir John Tooke in 2008, after the emergence of failings and scandals surrounding specialty training recruitment through its online application process: Medical Training Application Service (MTAS). Prior to MMC, entry into specialist surgical training was through a selection system organised by the medical deaneries. For example, entry into general surgical specialist training required meeting set criteria specified by the deanery, such as passing the Membership of the Royal College of Surgeons (MRCS) surgical exam, writing a number of first author publications, evidence of research skills (e.g. a Master's degree or Ph.D.). Importantly, surgical mentors had the ability to support their candidates directly, by writing glowing references or using their personal contacts with the selection team.

However, under MTAS, all specialist training posts would be advertised under a centralised scheme which did not permit the 'biased' interventions of surgical mentors. It is this pivotal change in the application process, whereby personal recommendations from consultants who have worked with candidates cannot influence a trainee's entry into a training programme, that Scarlett (see Section 6.3) bemoans. Instead, points are allocated to each trainee depending on how well they meet the selection criteria, which has led to shortlisted candidates competing against each other in an OSCE.[2]

However only 18,500 training posts were available for 32,000 applicants, which meant that over 14,000 junior doctors were left without training jobs (Tooke 2008). Scarlett and a few other of my interviewees are members of this 'lost tribe' of doctors who could not be placed in training programmes. Concerns were expressed that without the prospect of training positions, medical trainees would either seek employment abroad or leave medicine altogether (Shannon 2007; Gordon 2007). Large protests and rallies were held across the country, with doctors striking and marching against MMC and MTAS (Delamothe 2007; Boseley 2007; Eaton 2007).

The introduction of the 48-hour work week, or, European Working Time Directive (EWTD), was rolled out to hospitals across the UK at the same time. Doctors' Unions and the British Medical Association (BMA), alike, voiced concern that to be compliant with the reduced work hours, hospitals would have to recruit extra doctors into service jobs that carried no training prospects or career progression, thus creating, '*a permanent subclass of cheap, undertrained sub-specialists*' (Brown et al. 2007).

The Tooke inquiry was highly critical of MMC, stating that it had been an 'overambitious' strategy which had not engaged with the medical profession regarding how the recruitment process should be instituted or structured (Tooke 2008). These findings were supported by the review organised by the House of Commons Health Committee (2008). Following a judicial review of MTAS, brought about by pressure from Remedy UK (a junior doctors union), the application system was turned over from the Department of Health to the Royal Colleges and the national deaneries, who had, up until then, been responsible for the recruitment and training of all trainees. However, the concepts introduced by MMC were here to stay and continued to cause stress and anxiety for medical trainees in the UK. Scarlett's story illustrates these issues.

6.5   Women surgeons

The introduced complications to Scarlett's training path, brought about through the implementation of MMC, have only exacerbated the challenge of retaining women (like Scarlett) in surgical training and, idealistically, reducing the gender gap in this field.

In 2016, UCAS (the universities and colleges admissions service) reported that 58% of candidates accepted onto medicine and dentistry programmes in the UK were women. In 2018, 36% of consultants were women, although in surgery that figure is 12.2% in England (up from 3.3% in 1991 and 11.1% in 2011; RCS 2011, 2018). Thus, there is an evident discrepancy between the numbers of women who go into training and who subsequently become consultants. A number of factors may be implicated in this, including women more frequently choosing to work flexibly in order to dedicate more time to raising a family. This lengthens one's time spent training. Women trainees are present in all ten surgical specialties. In 2018, 27% of surgeons in England were identified as female compared with 24% in 2009 (NHS Digital 2018; Moberly 2018).

In July 2014, The Royal College of Surgeons of England, for the first time, appointed a female orthopaedic surgeon, Clare Marx, as the president of the college. The RCS commissioned research conducted by Exeter University that suggested that the low numbers of women in surgery was not due to a lack of ambition or reluctance to the long work hours, but rather to a perception held by women that they were unlikely to succeed comparable to their male counterparts (RCS 2014a).

6.6 The 'good trainee'

Scarlett believes that the characteristics of a 'good doctor' must be evident in any candidate applying for a place on a surgical training scheme. Therefore, she judges the new system of training on how well it identifies and distinguishes 'good' trainees. This notion of 'goodness' appears to be what controls and regulates the *visibility* of a trainee, for Scarlett. In other words, whether a candidate has the qualities Scarlett associates with 'goodness' determines their legitimacy as a serious candidate for training. As discussed earlier, in using these narratives I am not concerned with veracity or the establishment of an 'objective truth'. Foucault rejects contemporary notions of 'truth' and 'reality' as formed by the dominant opinions of a given era. Instead, he focuses on how our stories ('fictions') create the reality that we live and believe in and thus constitute what we conceive to be 'true'.

Scarlett understands that MMC aspired to eradicate the inequities inherent in the old system ('at least it's not as nepotistic as it used to be'). However, she believes that she was successful in the older system, that is, she was recognised as a good trainee and promoted because of her hard work and conscientiousness. These attributes were recognised by her supervising consultants as evidence that she had the intrinsic qualities necessary to be a 'good doctor'. I asked Scarlett to describe what she meant by a 'good trainee/doctor':

(If) you were to ask people who were assessing me to ask why they think I'm a good doctor, and they mostly think I am, they would say that it's because I am dedicated, I'm a good team player, I work hard, I have fun at work, and those are all true things. I really do love being there and the team atmosphere.

Within the older system, favoured by Scarlett, 'good trainees' were identified through inherent abilities, which are demonstrated in the cooperative relations established in work communities. Scarlett firmly believes that these qualities are intrinsic to individuals (e.g. dedication and diligence must be present before entry into a training programme). It is not the task of training systems to instil these qualities. One either has these traits or not. A community of peers and seniors, within the older system, provided unofficial (non-electronic/non-paper) assessments on a trainee's performance at work. Trainees who were 'not up to par' did not progress because they lacked the recognition and support of senior surgeons. This judgement of trainees was based on what Scarlett terms 'human understanding': a senior surgeon's personal experience and knowledge of what a specific trainee was capable of in terms of her inherent abilities and work ethic. The absence or possession of these qualities regulated the visibility of trainees in the pre-MMC system. These themes echo the work of Lave and Wenger (1991), who wrote extensively on how learning (and advancement of learning) is intimately connected to processes of participation in a community of practice.

But Scarlett is critical of how the notion of goodness, a complex concept, is captured by the current (MMC-inspired) system of training:

> Let's say you've got five junior doctors . . . they are with our department for four months each . . . they are on-call with different people, they are on different wards all the time. . . . If at the end of that four-month block, you asked all the surgeons to put in order, the best to worst junior doctor . . . I suspect that they would pick the same order of doctors. And that's because you know [who's good] when you work with somebody. I suppose it's because you know your expectation of yourself. It takes a very short time to say, 'you know what? That person is extremely dedicated, they know their stuff, they've seen their patients, they're aware of everything that's going on, that's the junior doctor I would pick for my team'. . . . The question is how can you get that fact, into some kind of numerical scoring system. And the answer is, that it's very, very, very difficult to do, because once you start trying to put it in parameters, and make it all formal . . . you just can't do it.

Scarlett describes how the attitudes and aptitudes associated with a 'good trainee' make him an appealing member of the wider team and also regulate the visibility of that trainee. However, she concludes that capturing these characteristics, which are immanent to daily encounters of practice, is nearly impossible within the current assessment format, which relies on a numeric system of categories. I suggest that the unofficial, person-to-person assessments of performance (i.e. as opposed to the established assessments) better appreciate 'intra-actions' (Barad 2007) in practice: the layers of complexity involved in a surgeon's performance. Examples of intra-actions include the complex relations that form between a trainee's aptitude and attitudes, societal expectations of the trainee, the ethos of the hospital, the culture of the workplace and the facilities and equipment available to the surgeon. The newer system of training may struggle to recognise and accommodate these complex tiers of practice through a stringent application of a limited numerical system (Hodges et al. 1999; Van der Vleuten 2012; Pangaro and Ten Cate 2013).

In the pre-MMC era, competence was a function of how a trainee's abilities were informally rated by those who worked closest and alongside them (i.e. their peers and senior colleagues) (Sinclair 1997; Watt et al. 2008; Carracio and Englander 2013; Sambrook 2014). Whereas in the post-MMC training system, with its emphasis on *competency-based training*, the opinions and judgements of surgeons cannot contribute in the previous manner. The locus of the power relations has shifted. Systems of learning objectives and assessments, devised and influenced by various stakeholders (e.g. the GMC, the Department of Health, the Academic Royal Colleges), have replaced the personal evaluations provided by senior surgeons working in a community of practice (Norris 1991; CanMEDS 2000; De Cossart and Fish 2005; ACGME 2007). It may seem that what is being measured and judged is the actual capacity of an individual (or organisation) to perform. However, in reality, what is being evaluated is not the inherent ability of an individual but rather how closely the individual's performance meets the pre-defined criteria of the performative technology. In short, a trainee is assessed on how well she adheres to the pre-approved criteria being monitored and measured.

I suggest that Scarlett's narrative draws attention to the perceived inequities and injustices of the selection system for surgical training. Namely, the inherent abilities of a candidate, which are desirable and necessary to provide appropriate patient care (e.g. a sense of professional responsibility or duty), are identified and supported within human relationships in the workplace. These human relations, which Scarlett believes are critical to any process of selecting 'good trainees', have been replaced in favour of impersonal categories of performance. Such are not supported by human evaluations that could provide context and proof of the candidate's worthiness for selection. The question then arises as to what the trainer's role is in this system of competency-based assessments? Certainly, the assessments require observation and interpretation by a surgical trainer to ascertain whether the trainee has met the criteria being tested. But how are trainers empowered by the assessment format to generate evaluations of performance? Is there consistency between what a trainer identifies as important in a learning encounter and what is deemed relevant by established structured assessments? These are some of the issues I investigate in the next chapter. To return to Scarlett, she was eventually selected for a training programme, but her subsequent experience of training practices only validated her initial views. I revisit her experiences in the final chapter of this section.

6.7　Amy's story

There is so much focus by the government on outcomes, so we have to show the effect. We know there is a positive impact by using these workshops but you have to prove that patients are safer for it, so it's hard to demonstrate the value of it. That's the context and the framework that we're all thinking with now because that's how people are being judged. We do struggle with this on our courses, we struggle with measuring impact. You're talking about two days out of someone's annual schedule (spent on a course), how do you measure whether this is what's made the difference or not?

We're reluctant to just be seen as a course provider, we'd like education to mean something a bit broader for people coming to the college. Not just training. A bit more of everything really . . . all sorts of different types of education . . . more networking forums and less formal things, some e-learning that would be free, just a bit more investment is needed. We have a huge number of faculty who teach our courses and to be able to do a bit more with them as a community would be quite good.

I understand the importance of patient safety. But if you're going to value outcomes more than people, then you're stuck, aren't you? I'm not going to convince anybody by saying, "well, you'll have less trainees who are struggling." But how do I prove that or who cares if I prove that? If we had this (other forms of education) and surgeons reflected more then they might feel better coming to work every day, in which case I presume it will impact on how patients experience treatment. But how do you show that?

Amy, an educator at the Royal College of Surgeons (RCS), is involved in developing new training courses and modifying existing programmes. She vocalises how government strategies to prioritise and assure patient safety have challenged the activities of the College. As discussed earlier, serious investigations into the failings of healthcare have reconfigured medical services and training around an agenda of patient safety (Francis 2013; DOH 2014a, 2014b; GMC 2013; RCS 2014b). All organisations and personnel involved in medical education and training are required to demonstrate clear outcomes that link a particular clinical activity with the prioritisation and promotion of patient safety (GMC 2016).

Amy and the College education staff believe in the additional value of providing a broader portfolio of surgical education to accommodate the potential for change in both the role and identity of future surgeons. This includes efforts to support how surgeons conceptualise their professional practice along complementary pathways, such as networking events, e-learning and faculty development, as well as incorporating trainings that recognise the impact of technology on the profession. However, according to Amy, these forms of education are considered less important than the more established methods of training, such as anatomy courses or suturing classes. These latter courses are viewed as supportive of the patient safety agenda because they cultivate knowledge and skills linked to a surgeon's technical proficiency.

By contrast, non-traditional educational programmes, which target aspects of practice that may potentially make surgeons 'feel better about coming to work every day' (Amy's words), are not recognized, promoted or supported in similar ways. Examples of these forms of education include discussion forums or support groups that provide opportunities to exchange thoughts and ideas around events of practice. Why might this be? The emotional wellbeing of a clinician is a complex and nebulous concept, making it nearly impossible to measure and equally difficult to assess accurately and consistently. Such poses a major challenge for the current system of professional regulation, which largely relies on demonstrable outcomes. In these instances, the College is required to provide clear evidence demonstrating how attention to the emotional wellbeing of a surgeon could improve or strengthen the patient safety agenda, mandated by national policy. Identification of concrete, replicable outcomes to establish a connection between the affective state of a surgeon and the safety of patients is an enormously difficult task given the abstract and obscure nature of the relation. But does that make attempting to address the affective states of surgeons, as a pedagogic concern, an irrelevance?

6.8 Forms of learning that arise from the immanence of practice

I am not questioning the importance of theoretical knowledge or procedural skill, both of which constitute established mandatory training, nor its promotion over and above other aspects of learning and training. Instead, I draw attention to those *forms of learning* that are either neglected or 'lost' when mandatory knowledge and skills are developed in ways that totalise the nature and content of training. This is the dominant theme that emerges from Amy's analysis of the state of formal surgical training and education. To unpack her thoughts and ideas further, I have looked at Gilbert Simondon's writings on hylomorphism (Simondon 1964), first discussed in the earlier theoretical chapters.

The predefined outcomes that are mandated by NHS policy contribute to a form of governance and represent a hylomorphic scheme of training. This is unavoidable when organizing a system in which the transmission of the fundamental skills and knowledge associated with safe and proficient practice must be ensured. However, a hylomorphic framework of training risks overlooking *forms of learning and their respective modes of governance which arise from encounters* with actual clinical practice. Crucially, learning that emerges in these unforeseen and unpredictable ways are associated with how the clinical problem comes to be a matter of concern and interest for the clinician. It signifies how clinical learning 'in the field' can become meaningful, as well as potentially transformative for existing practice.

Brian Massumi (2009), when commenting on Simondon's theory, distinguishes those aspects of learning that arise from the experience of being immersed in an event of practice (and which are therefore inherent to this specific encounter) as a 'form taking activity' (Massumi et al. 2010, p. 43). This concept resonates with Michael Polanyi's (2009) writings on tacit knowledge, as well as with Donald Schon's (1983) theory of knowing-in-action. Separately, knowledge that is assimilated from official manuals of training reflect learning that Massumi identifies as a 'form taking passivity'. I suggest that the learning which emanates from a *form-taking activity* can *transform* a physician's practice in two important ways.

First, such extends what is already known for both learner and teacher by way of creating additional knowledge and skills beyond the subject matter being taught/learned. Second, the novel ways of thinking and doing that emerge from being immersed in actual clinical encounters can also modify existing foundational practices of knowledge and skill, so as to ensure that these remain current and practically applicable.

An example of a form-taking activity yielding benefits is the development of laparoscopic surgery (keyhole surgery). This minimalist technique, which avoids large incisions and gross dissections, initially arose in the field of gynaecology. However, surgeons discovered that the technique could be applicable in other disciplines of surgery, such as colorectal and hepatobiliary surgery. This development represents an *extension of the technique* by creating novel methods to manipulate the procedure more widely. But the development of laparoscopic surgery also led to a modification in the principles of generic surgical practice.

Laparoscopic incisions are smaller, involve less dissection and are not as invasive as standard surgery. The technique is associated with quicker recovery times and less post-operative pain (Veldkamp et al. 2005; NICE 2006; Papadima et al. 2009; Varela et al. 2010). As a consequence, patients require less analgesia, mobilise quicker and discharge home sooner, frequently returning to work sooner (Burns et al. 2010; Hayden 2011). For instance, patients undergoing a laparoscopic removal of their gallbladder (one of the most common routine surgeries in the UK) are advised that they can be discharged home the same day of the surgery and can expect to return to work within two weeks or sooner.

Laparoscopic surgery is a remarkable advancement from the days when a gallbladder was extracted through a large incision in the abdomen that necessitated at least four weeks of recovery time, and which brought considerable post-operative pain. This patient experience demonstrated to surgeons the benefits of making surgery minimally invasive, leading to a modification of generic surgical practice. It is also an example of the reinforcing causality that occurs between how humans think about technology and how technology can, in turn, alter what society considers to be well established 'norms'. That is, in this scenario, specifically, surgeons contemplated using advances in surgical technology to minimise the trauma from surgery. The resulting improvement in recovery for patients challenged historic perspectives about how patients should feel after surgery, for example debilitating pain from big incisions became both unacceptable and wholly undesirable.

6.9   Expanding the 'capacities' of a surgeon

In her interview, Amy discusses professional development beyond mandatory training, wherein surgeons can contemplate aspects of their practice unencumbered by the outcomes agenda. Such opportunities can present surgeons with a *space* to think critically, without constraints, and about how their practice *matters* to them. Amy proposes that such opportunities may contribute to improving the patient experience. This objective closely parallels the aims of reflection-in-action: recalling practice in contemplative ways. However, notable differences exist. First, reflective practice as presented and promoted by both the GMC and the training deaneries encourages 'standing apart' from an event, in order to maintain an objective position (which is also dispassionate and logical) when reviewing an experience or encounter. Second, the perception and the enactment of reflection are framed as rational exercises. That is, the thoughts and actions that emerge through the experience are largely considered as cognitive processes.

John Dewey (1933) described reflection as an 'active, persistent, and careful consideration of any belief or supposed form of knowledge in the light of the grounds that support it and further conclusions to which it tends' (p. 9). But, as discussed in earlier chapters, I have hypothesized that the initial impact of an encounter is first affective and prior to cognitive processes intervening. How, then, do we reflect rationally on a phenomenon that is intangible and non-visible, manifesting prior to consciousness? I do not believe that there is one firm solution to this question. In fact, there cannot be if one subscribes to the ideas advocated in this book which first recognises the individual and unique nature of singular encounters with practice. Instead, what I have attempted to do is illuminate the affective complexities of practice, probing its nature and querying the resultant effects.

Contemplating these aspects of practice, which are non-rational and non-conscious can help make explicit what motivates, drives and shapes the ways in which clinicians think, see, understand and act. As educators, the main goal is to try to draw alongside these affective encounters of learning and practice in an effort to sympathise, support and understand how such ideas and intensities of experience connect the learner/practitioner to the event.

In summary, Amy's narrative calls for a coherence between how something in practice matters to a surgeon and the regulatory demands of healthcare. A collaborative bridging of the two has the potential to generate conditions that create enduring values in clinical practice, including candour, compassion and competence.

> The obligations and challenges of candour serve to remind us that for all its technological advances, *healthcare is a deeply human business*. Systems and processes are necessary supports to good, compassionate care, but they can never serve as its substitute. It follows from this that *making a reality of candour is a matter of hearts and minds* more than it is a matter of systems and processes, important as they can be. *A compliance-focused approach will fail* . . . systems and processes can only serve to structure a regulatory conversation about compliance. The commitment to candour has to be about values and it has to be rooted in *genuine engagement of staff*, building on their own professional duties and their personal commitment to their patients.
>
> (RCS 2015, p. 17, my emphasis)

This quotation is taken from *Building a Culture of Candour* (RCS 2015), a report commissioned by the then health secretary, Jeremy Hunt, and which was precipitated by the investigation into unacceptable standards of patient care at Mid Staffordshire NHS Trust (Francis 2013). The authors of the report rightly state that a culture of transparency is only possible if there is actual staff *engagement* with practice over and above the effects of regulatory mechanisms.

6.10   Outcomes and measuring performance

Amy's narrative highlights the challenges created by the adoption of an outcomes-driven agenda in surgical education and training. Strong parallels can be drawn here with the performative outcomes agenda in school education. On this topic, the writings of Stephen Ball (1997, 2003, 2013, 2015), which are critical of attempts to quantify and measure aspects of performance for both learners and teachers, help elucidate this matter. I use Ball's notion of 'performativity' to extend the initial arguments I raise in the earlier analysis of Amy's narrative.

> Performativity is a technology, a culture and a mode of regulation that employs judgements, comparisons and displays as means of incentive, control, attrition and change – based on rewards and sanctions (both material and symbolic). The performances (of individual subjects or organisations) serve as measures of productivity or output, or displays of 'quality', or 'moments' of promotion or inspection. As such they stand for, encapsulate or represent the worth, quality or value of an individual or organisation within a field of judgment. The issues of who controls the field of judgments is crucial. . . . Who is it that determines what is to count as a valuable, effective or satisfactory performance and what measures or indicators are considered valid?
>
> (Ball 2003, p. 216)

'Performativity', a term initially introduced by Jean-Francois Lyotard (1984), is suggested by Ball (2003) to be one of three policy technologies (the others being 'the market' and 'managerialism') in educational reform. He argues that performance, itself, is judged and compared so that it comes to represent the 'worth' of the individual or organisation. In other words, the performance totalises the contribution made by the individual/organisation. Ball problematises the way in which categories of judgements are established by asking *who determines which criteria are deemed valuable and which are not*? Amy's narrative emphasises this struggle. What she personally believes to be beneficial and valuable to the professional development of surgeons (gathered from her experiences of training surgeons) is obscured by what is formally identified in policy text as worthy and effective. Performativity is construed through what appears to be a rational and objective lens. That is, it creates fixed outcomes of performance that demonstrate the prioritisation of patient safety. However, as she opines, it is very difficult to reduce the complexity of a surgeon's affective state to simple categories that are amenable to assessment.

Ball describes how government discourses of performativity subjectivise teachers in specific ways, so that reform is instituted beyond structural organisations to include human subjects (teachers). In order to be considered a good and effective teacher, according to such discourses, one must be able to define one's professional identity within the associated concepts and language, such as 'producers/providers' or 'managers'.

> New roles and subjectivities are produced as teachers are re-worked as producers/providers, educational entrepreneurs and managers and are subject to regular appraisal and review and performance comparisons. We learn to talk about ourselves and the relationships, purposes and motivations in these new ways.
>
> (ibid., 218)

This framework of values focuses on prescribed identities of performance. *The Standards for Surgical Trainers* (2014), produced by the Royal College of Surgeons of Edinburgh (RCSE), illustrates these important points well. This document was produced as part of a wider initiative to formally recognise surgical trainers through a process of training and accreditation. Today, all surgeons engaged as surgical teachers must register their role with the GMC and produce the relevant documentation to support their claim.

I now draw attention to this document's introduction of two particular categories used to distinguish groups of teachers (see Figure 6.1): the 'effective trainer' versus the 'excellent trainer'. The document identifies the *effective trainer* as displaying behaviours that are easily demonstrable (RCSE 2014, p. 7) in clinical practice. Whereas, the *excellent trainer* is defined as engaging in teaching activities that go beyond the clinical workplace; engaging with training activities that improve overall patient safety, developing research projects and promoting the widespread use of mandated assessment procedures. These examples of 'excellent' behaviour reflect the wider agenda of professional regulation that has been predominantly spearheaded and promoted by the DOH and GMC, evidenced by the principles of *Good Medical Practice* (2013).

The difficulty arises when other forms of surgical teaching emerge from actual learning encounters in clinical practice, such being neither formalised by the trainers' guide nor reflective of the discourse on performativity. These forms of teaching and learning (i.e. surgical pedagogies) represent *adventures of pedagogic work* – they exceed attempts to predefine how trainees and trainers identify and perform in actual incidences of practice. By going further, these *immanent pedagogies* explore ways of trying to capture and understand what matters for learners, a population with eclectic modes of optimal learning.

Framework Area 5:
Supporting and monitoring educational progress

As a trainer you are able to set appropriate goals and review your trainee's progress in regard to these and the agreed curriculum.

The Effective Trainer

A. Sets an appropriate learning agreement with the trainee that complies with current curriculum stage.
B. Reviews and monitors the trainee's progress though regular meetings.
C. Uses e-portfolios (e.g. ISCP) to monitor the trainee's progress.
D. Provides written structured reports on the trainee's progress.
E. Identifies and engages with the trainee in difficulty.

The Effective Trainer

F. Engages in research, development and governance activities in the wider surgical training context.
G. Provides coaching and mentoring for trainees beyond basic requirements.

Framework Area 6:
Guiding personal and professional development
As a trainer you are able to act as a role model and source of guidance in the wider sphere of professionalism in the surgical workforce.

The Effective Trainer

A. Demonstrates exemplary professional behaviour.
B. Builds effective supervisory relationships balancing confirmation with challenge.
C. Sets and maintains personal and professional boundaries when supervising trainees as laid out in Good Medical Practice.
D. Identifies the need for careers or personal advice or support (e.g. occupational health, counseling, deanery careers unit) and refers on to other agencies in a timely manner.

The Effective Trainer

E. Is involved in the wider context of professional development of trainees
F. Develops skills related to coaching and mentoring above the standard supervisory role.

Framework Area 7:
Continuing professional development as a trainer
As a surgical trainer you continuously review and enhance your own performance as a trainer.

The Effective Trainer

A. Gathers feedback on their own performance as a trainer to benchmark against training curriculum.
B. Acts to improve their performance as a trainer.
C. Maintains up to date professional practice in all contexts in keeping with the principles of Good Medical Practice.

The Effective Trainer

D. Actively challenges poor practice and champions positive change in themselves and others.
E. Engages in further self-development as a trainer and promotes development in others.

Figure 6.1 Core and desirable skills and attributes of an 'effective trainer' versus an 'excellent trainer'.
Source: (RCSE 2014, p. 10).

Notes

1 MMC – Modernising Medical Careers was a controversial postgraduate medical training programme introduced in 2005 in the UK. It replaced the original system of training grades and introduced routine assessments of skills and activities. The independent review of MMC by Prof. John Tooke strongly criticised the way in which the programme was instituted, highlighting the inadequacies and inefficiencies of the system.
2 OSCE or objective structured clinical examination is a performance-based test of candidates through a series of stations which allows evaluation of clinical skills, decision-making and judgement skills, practical skills and knowledge. Candidates are set specific tasks at each station and assessed through direct observation of behaviour.

References

Accreditation Council for Graduate Medical Education (ACGME). (2007). "General Competencies." In *Outcome Project*. Chicago, IL: ACGME.

Albanese, M., Mejicano, G., et al. (2008). "Defining Characteristics of Educational Competencies." *Medical Education*, 42: 248–255.

Ball, S. J. (1997). "Policy Sociology and Critical Social Research: A Personal Review of Recent Education Policy and Policy Research." *British Educational Research Journal*, 23 (3): 257–274.

Ball, S. J. (2003). "The Teacher's Soul and the Terrors of Performativity." *Journal of Education Policy*, 18 (2): 215–228.

Ball, S. J. (2013). *Foucault, Power and Education*. New York and London: Routledge.

Ball, S. J. (2015). "What Is Policy? 21 Years Later: Reflections on the Possibilities of Policy Research." *Discourse: Studies in the Cultural Politics of Education*, 36 (3): 306–313.

Barad, K. (2007). *Meeting the Universe Halfway: Quantum Physics and the Entanglement of Matter and Meaning*. Duke University Press.

Boseley, S. (2007). "Junior Doctors Driven Abroad by New System." *The Guardian*, 2 March. Retrieved from www.theguardian.com/society/2007/mar/02/health.politics1.

Brown, M., Boon, N., et al. (2007). "Medical Training in the UK: Sleepwalking to Disaster." *Lancet*, 369 (9574): 1673–1675.

Burns, E., Naseem, H., et al. (2010). "Introduction of Laparoscopic Bariatric Surgery in England: Observational Population Cohort Study." *British Medical Journal*, 341: c4296.

Butler, J. (1997). *The Psychic Life of Power: Theories in Subjection*. Stanford: Stanford University Press.

Butler, J. (2005). Giving an Account of Oneself. Fordham University Press.

Carracio, C. L., and Englander, R. (2013). "From Flexner to Competencies: Reflections on a Decade and the Journey Ahead." *Academic Medicine*, 88: 1067–1073.

CanMEDS. (2000). "Extract from the CanMEDS 2000 Project Societal Needs Working Group Report." Medical Teacher, 22: 549-54.

Davis, M. H., Ponnamperuma, G. G., and De Cossart, L. (2007). "Education in Surgery: Competency-Based Training." *The Bulletin of the Royal College of Surgeons of England*, 89 (10): 342–345.

DeCossart, L., and Fish, D. (2005). *Cultivating a Thinking Surgeon: New Perspectives on Clinical Teaching*. TFM Publishing Ltd.

Delamothe, T. (2007). "Why the UK's Medical Training Application Service Failed." *British Medical Journal*, 334: 543–547.

Department of Health. (1993). *Hospital Doctors: Training for the Future*. Working Group on Specialist Medical Training. London: Department of Health.

Department of Health. (1995). *Hospital Doctors: Training for the Future*. Working Group on Specialist Medical Training. London: Department of Health.

Department of Health. (2003). *Unfinished Business. Report of the Chief Medical Officer in England Setting Out Proposals to Reform the SHO Grade*. London: Department of Health.

Department of Health. (2014a). *Hard Truths, the Journey to Putting Patients First: Volume One of the Government Response to the Mid Staffordshire NHS Foundation Trust Public Inquiry*. Retrieved from www.gov.uk/government/uploads/system/uploads/attachment_ data/file/270368/34658_Cm_8777_Vol_1_accessible.pdf (Accessed 12 January 2016).

Department of Health. (2014b). *Introducing the Statutory Duty of Candour: A Consultation on Proposals to Introduce a New CQC Registration Regulation*. Retrieved from www.gov.uk/government/uploads/system/uploads/attachment_data/file/295773/Duty_ of_Candour_Consultation.pdf.

Dewey, J. (1933). *How We Think*. Mineola, NY: Dover Publications.

Eaton, L. (2007). "Junior Doctors Lobby MPs in MTAS Protest." *British Medical Journal*, 334 (7599): 871.

Foucault, M. (1972). *The Archaeology of Knowledge*. London: Routledge.

Foucault, M. (1975). Birth of the Clinic: An Archaeology of Medical Perception. New York, NY: Vintage.

Foucault, M. (1982). "The Subject and Power." *Critical Inquiry*, 8 (4): 777–795.

Francis, Sir Robert. (2013). *The Report of the Mid Staffordshire NHS Foundation Trust Public Inquiry. Executive Summary*. London: The Stationary Office.

General Medical Council (GMC). (2016). *Promoting Excellence: Standards for Medical Education and Training*. Retrieved from www.gmc-uk.org/Promoting_excellence_ standards_for_medical_education_and_training_0715.pdf_61939165.pdf.

General Medical Council. (2013). *Good Medical Practice*. London: General Medical Council.

Gordon, B. (2007). "How This Government Views Junior Doctors Has Left Me No Choice But to Move Abroad." *The Telegraph*, 27 July.

Hall, D. E. (2004). *Subjectivity*. Routledge.

Hayden, P. (2011). "Anaesthesia for laparoscopic surgery." Continuing Education in Anaesthesia, Critical Care & Pain, 11(5): 177-80.

Hodges, B., Regehr, G., McNaughton, et al. (1999). "OSCE Checklists Do Not Capture Increasing Levels of Expertise." *Academic Medicine*, 74: 1129–1134.

House of Commons Health Committee. (2008). *Modernising Medical Careers: Third Report of Session 2007–2008, Vol. 1*. London: The Stationary Office Ltd.

Lave, J., and Wenger, E. (1991). *Situated Learning. Legitimate Peripheral Participation*. New York: Cambridge University Press.

Lurie, S. J., Mooney, C. J., and Lyness, J. M. (2011). "Commentary: Pitfalls in Assessment of Competency-Based Educational Objectives." *Academic Medicine*, 86: 412–414.

Lyotard, J. F. (1984). *The Postmodern Condition: A Report on Knowledge*. Manchester: Manchester University.

Massumi, B., De Boever, A., et al. (2009). "'Technical Mentality' Revisited: Brian Massumi on Gilbert Simondon." Parrhesia, 7: 36-45. Retrieved fromhttps://www.parrhesia-journal.org/parrhesia07/parrhesia07_massumi.pdf

Massumi, B., De Boever, A., et al. (2010). "'Technical Mentality' Revisited: Brian Massumi on Gilbert Simondon." *Parrhesia*, 1 (7): 36–45.

Moberly, T. (2018). "A Fifth of Surgeons in England Are Female." *British Medical Journal*, 363: k4530.

NHS Digital. (2018). *Narrowing of NHS Gender Divide But Men Still the Majority in Senior Roles*. Retrieved from https://digital.nhs.uk/news-and-events/latest-news/narrowing-of-nhs-gender-divide-but-men-still-the-majority-in-senior-roles.

NICE (National Institute for Health and Care Excellence). (2006). *Laparoscopic Surgery for Colorectal Cancer*. Retrieved from www.nice.org.uk/guidance/ta105.

Norris, N. (1991). "The Trouble with Competence." *Cambridge Journal of Education*, 21: 331–341.

Pangaro, L., and Ten Cate, O. (2013). "Frameworks for Learner Assessment in Medicine: AMEE Guide No. 78." *Medical Teacher*, 35: 1197–1210.

Papadima, A., Lagoudianakis, E., et al. (2009). "Repeated Intraperitoneal Instillation of Levobupivacaine for the Management of Pain After Laparoscopic Cholecystectomy." *Surgery*, 146 (3): 475–482.

Polanyi, M. (2009). *The Tacit Dimension*. Chicago, IL: University of Chicago Press.

Royal College of Surgeons of Edinburgh (RCSE). (2014). *Standards for Surgical Trainers*. Retrieved from https://fst.rcsed.ac.uk/media/9403/surgical-trainers-lr.pdf.

Royal College of Surgeons of England. (2011). *Surgical Workforce 2011: A Report from the Royal College of Surgeons of England in Collaboration with the Surgical Specialty Association*. Retrieved from www.rcseng.ac.uk/surgeons/surgical-standards/docs/2011-surgical-workforce-census-report.

Royal College of Surgeons of England. (2014a). *Women Surgeon Statistics*. Retrieved from http://surgicalcareers.rcseng.ac.uk/wins/statistics.

Royal College of Surgeons of England. (2014b). *Good Surgical Practice*. RCSE: Professional Standards.

Royal College of Surgeons of England. (2015). *Duty of Candour: Guidance for Surgeons and Employers. RCS: Professional Standards*. Retrieved from www.rcseng.ac.uk/news/docs/1-duty-of-candour-web-final.pdf (Accessed 1 March 2016).

Royal College of Surgeons of England. (2018). *Statistics: Women in Surgery*. Retrieved from www.rcseng.ac.uk/careers-in-surgery/women-in-surgery/statistics/.

Sambrook, P. (2014). "The Nature of Surgical Education Early in the 21st Century." *Annals of Maxillofacial Surgery*, 4 (2): 125–126.

Schon, D. A. (1983). *The Reflective Practitioner*. London: Temple Smith.

Shannon, C. (2007). "MTAS – Where Are We Now?" *British Medical Journal*, 334: 824–827.

Simondon, G. (1964). *L'individu et sa Genese Physico-biologique*. Paris: Presses Universitaires de France.

Sinclair, S. (1997). *Making Doctors: An Institutional Apprenticeship*. Oxford and New York: Berg.

Smith, M. (n.d.). *What Is Pedagogy?* Retrieved from http://infed.org/mobi/what-is-pedagogy/.

Tooke, J. (2008). *Aspiring to Excellence: Findings and Final Recommendations of the Independent Inquiry into Modernising Medical Careers*. Retrieved from www.medschools.ac.uk/AboutUs/Projects/Documents/Final%20MMC%20Inquiry%20Jan2008.pdf.

Touchie, C., and Ten Cate, O. (2016). "The Promise, Perils, Problems and Progress of Competency-Based Medical Education." *Medical Education*, 50: 93–100.

Van der Vleuten, C. P. M. (2012). "The Assessment of Professional Competence: Developments, Research and Practical Implications." *Advances in Health Science, Theory and Practice*, 1: 41–67.

Varela, J. E., Wilson, S. E., and Nguyen, N. T. (2010). "Laparoscopic Surgery Significantly Reduces Surgical-Site Infections Compared with Open Surgery." *Surgical Endoscopy*, 24 (2): 270–276.

Veldkamp, R., Kuhry, E., et al. (2005). "Laparoscopic Surgery Versus Open Surgery for Colon Cancer: Short-Term Outcomes of a Randomized Trial." *Lancet Oncology*, 6 (7): 477–484.

Watt, I., Nettleton, S., and Burrows, R. (2008). "The Views of Doctors on Their Working Lives: A Qualitative Study." *Journal of the Royal Society for Medicine*, 101: 592–597.

7 Learner Identities

how is the surgical trainee characterised and regulated within clinical training materials?

This chapter examines how the trainee is represented (specifically, pedagogised) in teaching practices. It queries how pedagogic practices contained in the currently promoted surgical curriculum and workplace assessments *identify, position and regulate* learners (i.e. trainees) and teachers (i.e. trainers). By problematising the nature of training practices, that is, both the theoretical and the lived experience, I attempt to deepen the understanding of what factors and ideologies constitute how trainees and trainers are engaged in teaching and learning activities. How do the relevant training materials capture and accommodate the reality of clinical practice? This chapter begins with a short overview of the postgraduate training system and its components.

Postgraduate training, both in the UK and overseas, is structured on a model of competency-based medical education (CBME). The core curriculum comprises a series of competences to be identified in areas such as practical skills, behavioural attitudes and theoretical knowledge (e.g. physiology, pathology, etc.) (ISC 2016; RCPSC 2015). Trainees are evaluated at each stage of their training programme to ascertain whether acquisition of the necessary standard competences (associated with their particular level of training) has occurred. Assessments are also conducted for other specific areas, including operative ability, clinical judgement and decision-making skills.

The nature of surgical trainer involvement has changed markedly from the days of the apprenticeship system. It is now required that surgical trainees learn procedures in a stepwise fashion that facilitates the gradual acquisition of skill (ISC 2016) and, further, they are not expected to operate alone. Independent operating is permitted only upon a trainee demonstrating full competency in the relevant skills. Some of the criticisms levelled against CBME, and discussed in the previous chapter, include the following: the proposed shorter training periods make it more difficult to achieve competence and safety of practice, there is advocacy of reductionist approaches to practice and assessment, there is the potential for fostering a checklist attitude to complex clinical skills and there is a perception of competencies as discrete tasks, whereas actual clinical practice is entangled. Competency-based frameworks fail to fully capture all the knowledge, skills and abilities needed for safe practice. Accordingly, the current scheme of assessments does not adequately address all the competencies of a practicing physician.

7.1   Surgical training

Competency

With the aforementioned focus on the attainment of competency, it is important, first, to conceptualize what is meant by a competence:

> An observable ability of a health professional, integrating multiple components such as knowledge, skills, values, and attitudes. Since competencies are observable, they can be measured and assessed to ensure their acquisition.
>
> (Frank et al. 2010)

There are different levels of knowledge and skill that can, and should eventually, be reached within each competence. The objective is therefore to gradually increase one's competence level for each given skill. To use the example of haemostasis (simply put 'stopping bleeding'), a candidate will advance from knowing the basic concepts of haemostasis to a fluent practical application of this knowledge by demonstrating the ability to arrest bleeding in an actual clinical event. Attainment of a competence affirms that the student has met the necessary standard of practice and has demonstrated the expected 'outcome'. In addition, acquisition of competences at each stage of training determines whether or not a trainee may progress to the next stage of training in that specialty.

The Intercollegiate Surgical Curriculum Programme (ISCP)

The ISCP, first introduced in 2003, defines and establishes the pathway from Foundation Doctor to Consultant Surgeon in the NHS. It provides a specialty syllabus, assessment formats and a portfolio for junior doctors to record their activities, as well as a logbook to document their training operations.

The ISCP is an online resource through which one can access the relevant syllabus for each of the ten surgical disciplines: cardiothoracic surgery, general surgery, neurosurgery, Oral and Maxillofacial Surgery (OMFS), Otolaryngology (ENT), Paediatric Surgery, Plastic Surgery, Trauma and Orthopaedic Surgery (T&O) and Urology and Vascular Surgery. Prior to the introduction of the ISCP, there was both inadequately written documentation and also the lack of a general consensus on which theoretical knowledge and practical skills were required for a surgeon in training. 'What you needed to know for the job' was largely transmitted to trainees through the practical and oral tradition of apprenticeship training. In brief, the tradition of *apprenticeship* has pervaded surgical education for centuries and only been challenged as recently as the last two decades. During a period of apprenticeship, a surgical trainee was expected to learn by observation, assistance and eventually permitted to carry out procedures independently. The latter would often occur with no oversight or supervision, and it was not uncommon for the consultant trainer to not be physically present in the hospital while the trainee operated. The system was notorious for the indeterminate time spent in training.

The 1990s heralded the beginning of a period of transition in medical (surgical) education. The previously unquestioned structure of training (the apprenticeship system) and the indefinite training period were challenged. In 1992, Kenneth Calman, the then Chief Medical Officer, set up a working group. The aim was to bring postgraduate training in line with the requirements of the European medical directives (DOH 1993). The report proposed a streamlined specialist training programme with a defined curriculum and minimum training period. Successful completion of the postgraduate programme would result in formal qualification as a specialist in that particular field. This new training system was to be defined by clear educational objectives, training agreements and a move towards ensuring that trainees were competent, irrespective of how long they had spent in training (DOH 1995). A decade later, the introduction of the ISCP heralded a seismic change in training culture. One of the guiding principles of the curriculum programme was to make explicit the required knowledge and skills for surgical trainees.

How do surgical trainees progress through training?

Once a doctor is fully licensed to practice (i.e. following successful completion of foundation-years training), she then applies for entry onto core training in surgery. Following this, she decides which specialty within surgery she wishes to train in, and she applies for a place within it. Specialist training (ST years 3 to 8), comprises gradual acquisition of relevant skills within a particular surgical discipline (e.g. Vascular surgery or Orthopaedic surgery), with the ultimate goal of the trainee gaining qualification as a specialist in that discipline. For example, a core trainee (CT1 and CT2 – early years of surgical training) is expected to know the symptoms and management of acute appendicitis, whereas senior trainees (i.e. ST4 onwards) are expected to build on this knowledge toward an eventual demonstration of their ability to perform an appendicectomy (i.e. removal of the appendix), as well as their ability to successfully manage any complications that may arise from the surgery.

Specialist training begins at the designation of ST3 and completes at ST8. Progression from ST3 onwards depends on whether a trainee can demonstrate all the predetermined, necessary competences for ST3 level. The GMC sets the level or 'standard' it requires all trainees to achieve in their professional practice. The ISC then applies these standards to the content of the syllabus, dividing it into three components: theoretical knowledge, clinical and procedural skills and professional skills (ibid., p. 9–10). A trainee's level of theoretical knowledge of a given surgical topic is quantified using the following numerical scale:

1   Knows of
2   Knows basic concepts
3   Knows generally
4   Knows specifically and broadly

A similar numerical scheme is used for assessing the competence level of procedural and technical skill:

1   Has observed
2   Can do with assistance
3   Can do whole but may need assistance
4   Competent to do without assistance, including complications

A syllabus entitled 'professional behaviour and leadership skills' is also employed to itemise the appropriate behaviours and attitudes expected of trainees.

7.2   How is the trainee pedagogised within operative training practices?

The representations of the trainee (as a doctor, a learner, a carer and so on) involve relations of power that generate and mould particular kinds of subjects who think, learn and act in certain ways that reflect these relationships of power. Usher and Edwards (1994) have commented that: 'Power is manifested as relationships in a social network. . . . Power, through knowledge, brings forth active "subjects" who better "understand" their own subjectivity yet who in this very process subject themselves to forms of power' (p. 89). In this observation they draw attention to how certain types of knowledge are imbued with power, which creates specific pedagogic identities. To illustrate this idea, I look at how the surgical curriculum frames the technical skills necessary to perform a common training operation: the surgical repair of a groin hernia. Figure 7.1 illustrates the syllabus requirements for the procedure, that is, it identifies the levels of knowledge and skills expected at different stages of training: ST4 (two years of specialist training), ST6 (four years) and ST8 (near completion of training).

I draw the reader's attention to the yellow-highlighted text under the category of 'TECHNICAL SKILLS'. An ST4 trainee is expected to perform an entire hernia surgery with help from a trainer, who may offer verbal advice or assistance (level 3). Whereas an ST6 trainee is expected to both perform the procedure *without* trainer guidance or input (i.e. under similar expectations of a consultant surgeon), and also demonstrate the ability to recognise and manage any difficulties encountered during the operation. The syllabus identifies the 'need for (trainer) assistance' (ISC 2016, p. 10) as the following:

•   Can adapt to well-known variations in the procedure encountered, without direct input from the trainer.
•   Recognises and makes a correct assessment of common problems that are encountered.
•   Is able to deal with most of the common problems.
•   Knows and demonstrates when she needs help.
•   Requires *advice rather than help* that requires the trainer to scrub.

	ST4	ST6	ST8	Areas in which simulation should be used to develop relevant skills
ELECTIVE HERNIA				
OBJECTIVE				
Diagnosis + management, including operative management of primary and recurrent abdominal wall hernia				
KNOWLEDGE				
Anatomy of inguinal region including inguinal canal, femoral canal, abdominal wall and related structures e.g. adjacent retroperitoneum and soft tissues.	4	4	4	
Relationship of structure to function of anatomical structures.	4	4	4	
Natural history of abdominal wall hernia including presentation, course and possible complications	3	4	4	
Treatment options				
Current methods of operative repair including open mesh, laparoscopic mesh and posterior wall plication, to include the underlying principles, operative steps, risks, benefits, complications and process of each	3	4	4	
CLINICAL SKILLS				
Diagnose and assess a patient presenting with abdominal wall hernia, including inguinal, femoral, epigastric, umbilical, paraumbilical, rare hernias (such as obturator and Spigelian hernias) and incisional hernias	3	4	4	
Supervise the postoperative course in hospital and on follow-up	3	3	4	
TECHNICAL SKILLS				
Hernia repair-femoral	3	4	4	
Hernia repair-incisional	2	3	4	
Hernia repair-incisional recurrent	2	3	3	
Hernia repair-inguinal	3	4	4	Strongly recommended:
Hernia repair-inguinal recurrent	2	3	4	
Hernia repair-umbilical/paraumbilical	3	4	4	Strongly recommended:
Hernia repair-epigastric	3	4	4	Strongly recommended:

Figure 7.1 The competence levels in skills and theoretical knowledge required for general surgical trainees to perform hernia operations.

Source: (Intercollegiate Surgical Curriculum 2016, p. 83) Reproduced with permission from the RCSE.

These definitions suggest that a trainee in 'need for assistance' demonstrates a fluency and familiarity with the procedural theory, rationale and technical steps, whilst still requiring verbal or technical intervention from the trainer. These statements referring to the technical procedure identify the novice surgeon as a particular type of learner. The syllabus anticipates and establishes a specific trainee-skill relation based on chronological notions of competence. The trainee must first assimilate procedural theory and, second, achieve competent practice alongside the gradual withdrawal of trainer assistance or intervention. This particular representation of operative competence is well established, well accepted and is an extension of the historic tradition of the apprenticed surgeon. Competence is thereby conferred within this particular discursive practice.

My surgical colleagues may roll their eyes at this point, protesting that this is the 'natural' progression for achievement of proficiency – a stepwise acquisition of skill. It is not my intention to argue the merits or flaws of this learning methodology, particularly when it is a staple of my own practice as a trainer! Instead, what I wish to emphasise and draw attention to is how the established ways of 'doing things' are often cited as 'natural', 'obvious' or 'common sensical'. This uncritical and unquestioning approach can *obscure the power relations* that constitute this particular paradigm of operative surgery and which appear 'normal' or inevitable so that trainers and trainees submit to it, albeit unknowingly.

Why is this paradigm of operative practice problematic? First, the training operation (e.g. hernia surgery) is shaped, regulated and examined through this singular representation of surgery; there is an established and accepted order to learning an operation. All of this can serve to obfuscate a more comprehensive and effective approach (I argue) of identifying the trainee through other signifying practices. For example, what if a trainee demonstrates technical proficiency prior to assimilating the theoretical steps? What if the trainee displays fluency in the latter steps of the procedure prior to developing proficiency in the initial steps? On this point, Joseph, a consultant surgeon, describes later in this chapter how he needed opportunities to attempt specific parts of an operation in conjunction with or even prior to reading about the procedure before the theoretical knowledge made sense to him. In that circumstance, he argues, had he approached the relevant skill acquisition in the reverse, officially recognised order, he would have engaged in rote learning a procedure without assigning any meaning or relevance to it. He believes such to be suboptimal. Further to this point, there are certain trainees who may conceive of a procedure in ways that are neither stated nor approved by the transcendent frameworks of the curriculum. But when there is a singular, discursive approach to conducting a given operation, a trainee's effective modifications or self-discovered techniques, for example, may not be accommodated, even when such have been shown to be optimally successful or efficient.

A second major reason why this paradigm of practice is problematic concerns, specifically, the criteria for identifying competent operative practice. Despite appearing to do so, this criteria does not evaluate the *inherent* technical ability of the learner, herself, nor the learner's innate skill in performing the operation. The signifier of operative ability, which is marked as assimilation of knowledge and demonstration of independence from assistance, constructs the trainee and trainer as pedagogised subjects. That is, a learner's ability to operate is not viewed as an intrinsic capacity that can be discovered or developed, even though it appears that this is the objective of said surgical training. Instead, a trainee's inherent operative abilities are constituted exclusively through their adherence to specific training practices, which, in turn, create certain relations of power and governance that both shape and determine the subjectivities of a surgical trainee and trainer.

There is no doubt that complicated procedures require adequate trainer guidance to ensure the safety of the patient, whilst also teaching the learner appropriate technical methods. However, what I advocate is an *increased awareness* of how curricular strategies can mould training practices to exclusively reflect established components of skill considered critical by authorised bodies of training. These core skills, specified by the curriculum, evidently include incising and closing superficial tissues accurately, tying secure surgical knots and knowing the safe use of electrocautery (ISC 2016, p. 51). While proficiency in these techniques is crucial, the problem posed to a more comprehensive development of trainee, I argue, arises when a learner's identity as a competent surgeon is absolutely constituted and confined in terms of their ability to develop skills in these core elements; there is no room for exploring or recognising what inherent abilities they already possess.

In summary, we accept as reasonable and logical the current practice of surgical training (i.e. a trainee proceeds through a graded acquisition of skills toward an eventual independent competence for a given operation). Indeed, the subjectivities of both trainee and trainer emerge from submitting (unknowingly) to the forms of power and governance inherent in this conception of operative practice, and which also appear as obvious and natural. The difficulty arises when this particular discursive practice identifies surgical skill in a short-sighted manner that inhibits or neglects to acknowledge other representations or signifiers of technical skill. Such alternative representations may constitute how operative practice *matters* to trainees and, therefore, how forms of mattering may constitute personal forms of governance that affect how they learn. I expand this discussion further in the ensuing pages.

7.3   Thinking differently about operative training

> The point I wish to make is that you can't learn surgery by yourself. So, different people have different abilities to learn by watching, some people can repeat something after watching it once. I needed to first do things myself and figure it out in my head . . . because in my head I'm thinking there are many different ways that this could be done. . . . So, why would other ways not work and why must I do it this way only? Others don't think about the alternative ways of doing things.
>
> Most of our trainers are used to trainees who will carry out things in one approved way. But it can be a big advantage when doing difficult types of problems, because then your mind is attuned to looking at things from different angles and not necessarily using the one shot solution.
>
> (Joseph, Consultant Surgeon, London)

When I interviewed Joseph, he had been in his first consultant job for a few months. He works in a London teaching hospital at a tertiary specialist centre. 'What I am really in this job for is that I really like teaching. . . . For me that is the THE priority!' Joseph has specifically sought opportunities to train surgeons.

In his narrative, Joseph describes how trainees tend to adopt a singular approach when learning a new operation. The apprenticeship model of teaching operative skills was based on the premise that a student would learn from an expert surgeon by watching their operations, being instructed in that surgeon's particular way of 'doing surgery' and eventually emulating the surgeon's procedural techniques and practices. This model of surgical learning was premised on 'time spent in training'. The move to competency-based surgical training, however, shifted the emphasis of training away from time spent 'apprenticed' to a master surgeon towards demonstration of predefined competences in a procedure; "regulation of progression through training . . . [is] by the achievement of outcomes that are specified within the specialty curricula. These outcomes are competence-based rather than time-based" (ISC 2016, p. 4). However, I have queried whether this change, instead, reflects a move from a master surgeon towards a master (singular) method of practice. In other words, whereas previously a trainee would be expected to operate in the style of one trainer (therefore operating in one particular way), now a trainee is required to operate in a manner consistent with a single, predefined method that is recognised and reinforced by modern-day assessments.

Operative training relies on a transcendent framework of teaching: trainees are introduced to an established and historical tradition of technical skills. This involves following the approved format: steps of the procedure, shape of the incision and technique to dissect and handle tissues, for example. The operative method being learned is often an ancient discipline, and some techniques, for example trephining (i.e. making a hole in the skull, also known as a 'burr hole' in surgical parlance), have their origins in the neolithic period (Porter 1997). Another example is the technique of vascular anastomosis (i.e. joining two blood vessels together) developed by Dr. Alexis Carrel (1873–1944), for which he was awarded the Nobel Prize in 1912. Therefore, it is no surprise that techniques that have proved to be efficient, effective and to have 'stood the test of time' are unquestioningly taught and propagated in surgical practice. When faced with a novice surgeon, a trainer is therefore able to teach established and concrete technical skills (e.g. the 'best' way to tie surgical knots, the 'best' way to hold surgical instruments).

Joseph opined that these techniques form the building blocks of a surgical trainees' operative skill set. However, teaching traditional techniques should not limit an individual trainee's *process of discovery* in the operative field. But the dominant pedagogic approach in operative training can place too much emphasis on how to instruct and instil technical skills, whereby the resultant (even if unintentional) message is that skills can only be acquired through *unquestioned specific guidance*.

The reality is that nowadays, a trainee may rotate through a number of surgical jobs in which different expert surgeons are responsible for their operative training.

The trainee then learns from this collection of surgeons, each possessing their own interpretation of how best to perform an established technique (e.g. how to stop bleeding, how to sew vessels). During my own transplant training, every surgeon who instructed me in the technique of sewing blood vessels (i.e. vascular anastomosis) had a different take on the procedure. Each iterated the basic principles of the technique yet, in their effort to solidify their trainee's understanding, they each had their own interpretation of the nuances of the procedure, their own belief systems about why they did something in a particular manner and their own style of emphasis on certain components of the procedure. The benefit of a multi-surgeon teaching approach lies in the opportunity to learn different elements or 'tricks of the trade' from each trainer. Joseph firmly believes in the importance of having more than one way to approach a surgical problem. In turn, such permits trainees to develop a toolbox of operative techniques, based on what they have chosen to retain or discard from their training.

However, while the scope to pick and choose different operative styles or approaches is a definite advantage for a developing trainee, the reality in practice is different. That is, without concrete opportunities to attempt variations of a procedure in a safe and supervised environment that ensures patient safety, how do trainees discover what techniques, styles or approaches 'work' best for them? I suggest that it is through these opportunities to explore, which are not always adequately accommodated, that surgical trainees *discover practice*. Such a process of supervised discovery has significance for cultivating thoughtful and creative surgeons who can innovate in unfamiliar situations, specifically those that have not necessarily been iterated within official manuals of surgery. Joseph references this as problem solving 'in the field' when a surgeon is confronted by unfamiliar operative cases which cannot be resolved through an application of known or approved methods.

7.4 Expanding what operative training can be

Joseph's narrative raises three primary pedagogical objectives. The first concerns how trainees can be encouraged to expand their understanding of operative practice. Put another way, how can trainees be given some degree of freedom to explore Surgery so that they can create something new for themselves in terms of knowledge, skill or understanding, and that which exceeds what they have already been taught? There is also potential for these emerging capabilities to extend what is already known within the existing discipline of Surgery. This could lead to a contemplation of *what Surgery can become* or what it has the potential to achieve for both its community of surgeons as well as the greater public (i.e. beyond conceptualising Surgery through a collection of individual operations).

A second pedagogical objective raised by Joseph's narrative concerns what modes of thinking and being are important to cultivate an ability to cope with the immanence of surgical practice. That is, what attitudes and behaviours emerge from the thisness of surgical encounters and which are critical, therefore, to a surgeon's capacity to cope with the uncertainty of practice? Lastly, the third raised objective concerns how imagination and invention can be fostered while both maintaining the demands for patient safety and also meeting the criteria for competence. I have drawn on Gilbert Simondon's writings to explore these questions amidst an examination of the established norms and practices within surgical education.

This book advocates an approach to operative training that is open to the modes of thinking and doing that can arise within the uncertainty and haecceities of surgical practice. That is, I argue for a relaxation of pedagogic criteria and prejudgments on what training should be. Instead, embracing and incorporating this more open operative training is to support what a surgeon can *become* when encountering the immanence of practice. The notion of 'becoming', in simple terms, refers to *what can still be created in a situation rather than what already exists and is known*. Reconfiguring operative practice along notions of 'becoming' may lead to an enhanced understanding of what is *yet possible* in technical training. To explore this notion of 'what-is-yet-to-be' I turn to Simondon's concept of 'metastability' (1989): a state of limitless possibility or potential (Scott 2014). He conceives of individuals in terms of the relations that continually form and develop between what they are at a given moment and what can still be actualised in the present. This potential to develop into something new, which has previously not existed or come about, is the possibility inherent in a metastable system. A singularity such as an unanticipated event or encounter can disrupt this pool of potential and precipitate a process of 'individuation' to create a new state of being.

> The individual, then is always in relation to its milieu, which co-individuates along with it. As such the individual can never be considered as complete but always partial and in the process of individuation, the milieu always acting as a mediation between individual and world.
>
> (Mills 2016, p. 40)

Joseph, in his description of watching an operation as a trainee, discusses how he believes that, in certain circumstances, there are numerous ways to proceed in performing the given surgical operation:

> some people can repeat something after watching it once. I needed to first do things myself and figure it out in my head . . . because in my head I'm thinking there are many different ways that this could be done. . . . So, why would other ways not work and why must I do it this way only?

Although Joseph is aware of the potentialities that emerge from an encounter of observing someone else doing the procedure, he personally requires a broader application of 'doing by seeing'. What he is asserting, then, is the importance of opportunities to explore why that which he has been taught is condoned as the best way forward in a procedure. I suggest that what he is describing is his personal process of discovery, that is, how a particular technique or procedure comes to matter to him. It is not simply that he cannot learn from observing or from being instructed by a more experienced surgeon. I classify his thoughts as an illumination of the *necessary tension* that must exist between transcendent forms of learning (i.e. formal knowledge and skills) and the immanence of learning that arises from an application of transcendent practices.

Through a different but related consideration of this matter, I draw on Simondon's theory of metastability, which represents a pool of 'becoming'. That is, at any point in a procedure there is the potential for the surgery to unfold, or 'become', in a number of ways. The singularity that triggers an actualization of this metastable state (referred to by Simondon as 'dephasing') is the trainee being confronted by a technical problem in the procedure. For example, this may be an episode of unanticipated bleeding or an anatomical anomaly. It is in being immersed in the actual operative encounter of the surgery that the trainee has the opportunity to actualize the potentials that emerge from this encounter with practice. Through this adventure, he is able to derive meaning from the encounter. His practice comes to matter to him through this engagement, and he learns from the event. It may be that what he learns is an appreciation of why a procedure is conducted in a particular way. Equally, it is possible that he may discover a new way to resolve the technical difficulty, thus actualising a new potentiality.

What I assert through this analysis and application of Simondon's theory is that individuation provides the conditions of possibility for what operative knowledge can fully be for a given trainee, in addition to what already exists. Indeed, many training programmes have been built on systems of potentials that have contributed to the emergence of authorised practices and transcendent norms, thereby establishing what is known, how it is recognised and when it was approved. However, these systems of potentials, through the action of forming authorised norms, have too often come to be viewed as complete – meaning that there are no new or different ways to conceptualise a particular procedure or ways of training. But I argue that these structures and frameworks, in turn, also represent potentialities for further development in response to singularities that come from the environment.

Therefore, transcendent norms (familiar and established ways of doing things) are, 'in essence', metastable structures, which can be disrupted and disturbed by unanticipated or unfamiliar events in the operating theatre, to produce potentialities that act to create and expand how we think and practice in both surgery and surgical education.

7.5   Procedure-based assessment (PBA)

Procedure-based assessment (PBA) is an example of a workplace-based assessment (WBA) used to evaluate the development of operative skill. The WBAs were designed to investigate the knowledge, clinical skills, behaviour and attitudes of an individual in their relation to a particular medical procedure. WBAs are formative assessments, which are designed to provide feedback on performance in order to help trainees improve their familiarity with a procedure, as well as their proficiency and technique, so that they become expert and safe practitioners (Norcini 2003; Norcini et al. 2003; Norcini and Burch 2007; PMETB 2005; GMC 2010).

However, in recent years, WBAs (including PBAs) have come to represent examinations of performance and, as such, the formative feedback element has been misplaced (Norcini 2007; Phillips and Jones 2015). PBAs involve the trainer (assessor) conducting an observed assessment of the trainee performing a common ('index') operation in the speciality (e.g. a hernia repair). Figure 7.2 illustrate the three pages of the written format of the assessment. There are two principal components to the PBA. Each procedure is assessed via six 'domains' (i.e. consent, pre-operative planning and preparation, exposure and closure, intra-operative technique and post-operative management), each of which comprises its own criteria or 'competencies' to be met in order for a trainee to demonstrate successful completion of that stage, or, 'competent practice' therein. At the end of the procedure, the trainer must give an overall assessment of performance using a global assessment that features eight specific ratings. The highest rating reflects consultant-level practice.

PBAs utilise a didactic assessment format that itemises what must be observed (i.e. 'positive behaviours') at each step of the procedure. In addition, the trainer guidance specifies the *parameters* through which the 'positive behaviours' must be observed, such as through speaking or drawing:

The terms that form the assessment of the surgical procedure assert a *particular paradigm of operative practice*. In this paradigm, competence is conceived and framed through *physical expressions of practice* that are *visual*: the ability to demonstrate, supervise, vocalise, verbalise and mark out one's thoughts and actions at any given moment. It is through this discursive practice, which constitutes a 'physical' representation of operative surgery, that the surgeon becomes visible to both trainer and trainee. However, in this focus on demonstrable items, the assessment is therefore *not about inherent trainee ability*. I argue, then, that it is not a complete assessment of operative ability or clinical judgement *in* the trainee or *in* the surgical procedure, despite appearing to be so. Rather, the assessment discourse constructs, regulates and confirms a particular kind of surgical trainee within a specific pedagogic gaze.

Further, a significant danger inherent to PBAs lies in the fact that the dominant signifier of ability is *linguistic skill*. That is, to demonstrate that the required knowledge and skills have been assimilated and understood requires verbal expressions in this assessment format. Specifically, and when assessing surgical skill within this paradigm, the trainee's inherent capacity to perform a particular procedure is not considered as an innate skill that can be liberated or discovered. Instead, trainee ability is constituted in particular sites of practice, and this is done through verbal communication.

Critics may argue, 'how else are we to gather information on whether a trainee has the required knowledge to perform the procedure, if not by asking for an explanation?' I agree that this is a reasonable approach to take and one which offers the easiest method for ascertaining trainee understanding. However, it raises two issues. First, this method has been adopted as the exclusive form of expression of understanding. Second, in reality, surgeons adapt or adopt certain techniques of practice for a variety of reasons; like all human beings, they, too,

Your ratings should be judged against the standard for the Certification. Assessors are normally consultants (senior trainees may be assessors depending upon their training level and the complexity of the procedure)

IMPORTANT: The trainee should explain what he/she intends to do throughout the procedure. The Assessor should provide verbal prompts if required, and intervene if patient safety is at risk. A rating of Satisfactory can only be given if no prompting or intervention was required

Rating:
N = Not observed or not appropriate
D = Development required
S = Satisfactory standard for CCT (no prompting or intervention required)

Competencies and Definitions		Rating N/D/S	Comments about this section
II. Pre operation planning			
PL1	Demonstrates recognition of anatomical and pathological abnormalities (and relevant co-morbidities) and selects appropriate operative strategies/techniques to deal with these e.g. nutritional status		
PL2	Demonstrates ability to make reasoned choice of appropriate equipment, materials or devices (if any) taking into account appropriate investigations e.g. x-rays		
PL3	Checks materials, equipment and device requirements with operating room staff		
PL4	Ensures the operation site is marked where applicable		
PL5	Checks patient records, personally reviews investigations		
III. Pre operative preparation			
PR1	Checks in theatre that consent has been obtained		
PR2	Gives effective briefing to theatre team		
PR3	Ensures proper and safe positioning of the patient on the operating table		
PR4	Demonstrates careful skin preparation		
PR5	Demonstrates careful draping of the patient's operative field		
PR6	Ensures general equipment and materials are deployed safely (e.g. catheter, diathermy)		
PR7	Ensures appropriate drugs administered		
PR8	Arranges for and deploys specialist supporting equipment (e.g. image intensifiers) effectively		
IV. Exposure and closure			
EI	Demonstrates knowledge of optimum skin incision / portal / access		
E2	Achieves an adequate exposure through purposeful dissection in correct tissue planes and identifies all structures correctly		

Figure 7.2 Procedure Based Assessment (PBA) Form (ISC 2016) to assess an elective procedure: open repair of an inguinal (groin) hernia.

ITl (G)	Follows an agreed, logical sequence or protocol for the procedure		
IT2 (G)	Consistently handles tissue well with minimal damage		
IT3 (G)	Controls bleeding promptly by an appropriate method		
IT4 (G)	Demonstrates a sound technique of knots and sutures/staples		
IT5 (G)	Uses instruments appropriately and safely		
IT6 (G)	Proceeds at appropriate pace with economy of movement		
IT7 (G)	Anticipates and responds appropriately to variation e.g. anatomy		
IT8 (G)	Deals calmly and effectively with unexpected events/ complications		
IT9 (G)	Uses assistant(s) to the best advantage at all times		
IT10 (G)	Communicates clearly and consistently with the scrub team		
ITl1 (G)	Communicates clearly and consistently with the anaesthetist		
IT12 (T)	Carries out dissection purposefully and accurately to expose sac without compromising adjacent structures such as nerves and blood vessels		
ITl3 (T)	Identifies sac and assesses sac contents correctly		
IT14 (T)	Deals with sac contents appropriately by reduction / inspection / further procedure		
ITl5 (T)	Deals with sac appropriately by inversion / transfixion and excision		
ITl6 (T)	Completes a sound repair by an appropriate method without compromising adjacent structures		
VI. Post operative management			
PM1	Ensures the patient is transferred safely from the operating table to bed		
PM2	Constructs a clear operation note		
PM3	Records clear and appropriate post operative instructions		
PM4	Deals with specimens. Labels and orientates specimens appropriately		

Figure 7.2 Continued

PBA Details	
Emergency/Elective	[ ] Emergency [ ] Elective
Difficulty of procedure on this occasion	[ ] Easier than usual [ ] Average difficulty
	[ ] More difficult than usual
Performed in a simulated setting	[ ] Yes [ ] No
PBA performed while on a course	[ ] Yes [ ] No

Global summary		

Level at which completed elements of the PBA were performed on this occasion		Tick as appropriate
Level 0	Insufficient evidence observed to support a summary judgement	
Level Ia	Able to assist with guidance (was not familiar with all steps of procedure)	
Level Ib	Able to assist without guidance (knew all steps of procedure and anticipated next move)	
Level 2a	Guidance required for most/all of the procedure (or part performed)	
Level 2b	Guidance or intervention required for key steps only	
Level 3a	Procedure performed with minimal guidance or intervention (needed occasional help)	
Level 3b	Procedure performed competently without guidance or intervention but lacked uency	
Level 4a	Procedure performed uently without guidance or intervention	
Level 4b	As 4a and was able to anticipate, avoid and/or deal with common problems/complications	

Figure 7.2 Continued

can be guided by various and varying motivations. Observe this narrative which addresses the actions of practice by consultants in the field:

> I'm quite good at saying 'well, I don't understand that, what's your rationale, what's your surgical strategy?' Because at the beginning you think they just know everything and I don't understand. But because I've done the exam I know that they don't always (have a rational explanation based on theoretical knowledge). They do things a certain way because it's what they're familiar with, or because the patient lives in a sixth floor flat with his mum, or some other social thing which might have bearing on patient aftercare.
>
> (Eleanor, senior trainee, London)

Furthermore, the power implicit in this discursive practice (i.e. applying PBAs to surgical training) exerts inclusionary and exclusionary forces. The global rating assigned at the end of the assessment subjects the trainees to the gaze of certain knowledge and practice discourses by which their own practices have been

Table 7.1 Trainer Guidance.

TRAINEE COMPETENCIES	POSITIVE BEHAVIOURS
Communicates clearly with scrub team	Sets **positive tone** with appropriate greeting
Demonstrates careful skin preparation	**Supervises** painting of the operative field
Controls bleeding promptly by an appropriate method	**Responds** calmly by applying pressure
Follows an agreed, logical sequence for procedure	**Justifies** actions at any point in procedure
Achieves an adequate exposure through purposeful dissection/identifies all structures correctly	Gives a **running commentary** of the structures encountered
Demonstrates knowledge of optimum skin incision	**Verbally states** or **marks with a pen** anatomical landmarks

Source: (adapted from PBA Trainer Validation sheet p. 3, ISC 2016).

measured and categorised. In this evaluation, the signifier of ability is 'guidance'. Guidance is presented in a few different ways within the assessment, from the giving of advice, to guiding the trainee from a position as an assistant to the main surgeon in the procedure, to guidance as intervention when necessary or not. The provision and withholding of assistance by the senior person reflects the relations of power-knowledge that exist in the trainer-trainee relationship. Guidance appears to be required when a trainee is 'lacking' in knowledge or skill. For example, the Level 1a global score is defined as 'able to assist with guidance', further explicated as 'not familiar with all steps of the procedure'. Guidance, therefore, is equated here with 'help' or 'not familiar' (with the procedure, anatomy etc.).

Interestingly, guidance also appears to be implicated in the following assessment of a trainee, labelled as 3b and highlighted in yellow (see Figure 7.2): 'procedure performed competently without guidance or intervention but lacked confidence'. One might otherwise expect that demonstrating competence is automatically equated to being confident in performing the procedure. However, this assessment, in its language, adds a further tier to how competence is now understood. Specifically, it emphasises that demonstrating competence does not necessarily mean that the trainee has 'confidence'. But what is the motivation behind this differentiation? It's not clear whether the designation of 'confident' requires a trainer to make an assumption about the trainee's state of mind, or not. Scarlett makes the following comment:

> People say trainees develop at different times. I think that's only true partially because some people are just cocky and think they can do operations that they're really not fully trained to do. I remember this guy called Raj Pataki and they said to me, "how many hernias could you do?" And I said, "well, I could do one on my own, but I'm training and I therefore want somebody there who'll be able to tell me what I'm doing right and wrong." So they said, "ok, well, Raj could do it with you." I said, "well Raj has done 20 (hernia operations) and I've done 50! Raj is a cocky t*** and I'm a conscientious surgeon. That's the difference between us." So, I found it really frustrating

that they were like, "well, if you're a bit nervous take Raj with you." No! I'm not nervous, what I want is to improve every time I do this operation. It is a balance because at some point you just have to do it.

Scarlett highlights a particular difficulty often faced by capable yet conscientious trainees. Their reluctance to be used in the capacity of service providers for a hospital (in this case she was asked to do an operating list on her own to help reduce waiting lists) can be perceived as a lack of confidence. That is, colleagues, in their haste to address mounting service pressures, may rush to conclude that, as a senior trainee with sufficient experience, surely she should be comfortable and safe to operate independently. But, in reality, Scarlett views herself as a trainee who should continue to be guided and supervised. Such should be viewed as a highly desirable trait: a conscientious surgeon who understands her limitations and knows when to ask for help in the interest of prioritising patient welfare. The confidence of some of her colleagues, as she states so vividly in this excerpt, is not a demonstration of safe or competent practice but rather a reflection of their attitude and state of mind. Her comments emphasise the complexities involved in how 'skill' can be recognised and potentially misconstrued by trainees, trainers and non-surgical folk.

This example of a WBA demonstrates how notions of 'competence' are constructed around particular discourses of what is visible and measurable in practice. 'Competence' can be described as a *point de capiton*, a term introduced by Jacques Lacan (Zizek 1989, p. 101).

A *point de capiton* is an upholstery button which, once pinned down on a surface, causes folds of material to radiate from its centre. In the assessment discourses discussed, competence figuratively forms such a pin. Imagine that the assessments and conclusions made about a trainee radiate like the little lines of cloth made by the button. Where these lines converge is at the button, which signifies competence. This point of convergence enables everything that happens in this discourse on competence to be situated retroactively and retrospectively (Lacan 1993, p. 268). Another instance of such is the use of *patient safety* as a *point de caption* around which discourses on standards in practice, professionalism and regulation of trainees, for example, are configured.

Concluding thoughts on PBA assessment in surgical training

What is the purpose of instituting these assessments of practice, which have replaced the former, subjective evaluations of performance made by senior surgeons? Is it, as suggested by Scarlett earlier in the chapter, to remove perceived biases and prejudices and, thereby, foster a more equitable system? Further, whose interests are served in an '*a-subjective*' conception of assessment? Note that I have not described this system as 'objective' because my purpose is to emphasise the *absence of a surgeon's voice in this structure of assessment*.

I suggest that these post-MMC assessments, whilst described in the ISC as 'objective measures of performance', exist as subjective tools themselves, because they are constructed around what the official stakeholders in medical education collectively identify and believe to represent 'competence'. The narrative excerpts in this chapter exemplify the two conflicting discourses of competence in contemporary training. One has expectedly originated from diverse individuals being immersed in a community of, and reality of, surgical practice. Such is inevitably at odds with the second discourse, which arises from being evaluated by a 'dispassionate' and impersonal system of assessment. What distinguishes one discourse from the other is primarily the location of power in the assessment relationships. I now explore how forms of power manifest in training.

7.6   How do surgeons conceive practices of training?

Training is very much like apprenticeship isn't it. You're not really trained, you just follow people round and you take on as much as you do or don't. It's hard to quantify, it's hard to dispute whether it's a good way to train. My absolute favourite example of this is when I began Vascular surgery as a registrar (senior trainee) and I worked with Mark, who was my SHO (junior trainee). Mark had been an ST8 in cardiology (final year trainee prior to becoming a consultant) before joining my team. He got to the end of his cardiology training, he'd had kids and he thought, "you know what? I can't do this (cardiology) for my whole life." He retrained as a GP and in his GP training rotation he had come to vascular surgery to do a six-months placement.

His next training job as a GP was to be an SHO (junior trainee) in cardiology, based on the same ward that he had worked on as an ST8 in cardiology. So, he phoned up the deanery and said, "look guys, I was the ST8 on that ward and I've also just finished being the consultant for cardiology on that ward, so in terms of training, this placement is not going to be of any further benefit to me the six months I'm based there. And they said, "that's not true, because you'll learn completely different things being a junior on those wards." I mean, the mind boggles! And that's because it's some administrator who is just ridiculous. But he (Mark) thought, you know what, just sod it! He was just waiting out his three years training to be a GP and thought, "I'll do it, it'll be piss easy for six months!" He had tried to change it to something more useful, but they had refused.

(Scarlett, ST7 trainee)

7.7   The transcendence of training: 'becoming undone'

Scarlett uses the story of Mark to emphasise her view of relations in training, specifically those which contribute to how she constructs, first, herself (and Mark) as a particular kind of trainee and, second, the deanery as a particular authority of training (the trainer). Two specific pedagogic issues arise from this anecdote, which I wish to explore. The first concerns how Mark is told that, although he is a qualified expert in cardiology, he would still benefit from spending time as a trainee in that same specialty. What do these views communicate about how authority figures in training, such as the regional training deanery in this story, conceptualise and subjectivate trainees and learners? The second concerns that fact that Mark accepts this fate. What do such actions suggest about the nature of pedagogic relations in this encounter?

In this narrative, Scarlett describes the deanery as populated by 'administrators'. In other words, it is comprised of many non-medical folk who are unfamiliar or unaware of the realities of medical training, and who are primarily concerned with the practicalities of organising a training programme. As such, this training body categorises trainees according to established and approved criteria which are both rigid and fixed, and which create the norms used to evaluate trainees. Therefore, qualifications or experiences outside of this framework of norms are diminished or disregarded. These established, entrenched attitudes and behaviours of the training body indicate a 'transcendent organisation'. As already shown, a potential consequence of a transcendent approach is to conceive the trainee as uneducated or 'unknowing'. However, and also discussed earlier, these instances of 'unknowing' can present opportunities to interrogate what constitutes us. Namely, they allow for exploration of answers to such questions as, 'how are we constructed as learners and teachers', and what structures are in place to reinforce this particular configuration of subjectivities?

I begin to unpack, here, the two questions I raise at the beginning of this section. The writings of Judith Butler (2005) help to clarify key points I wish to make.

> Perhaps most importantly, we much recognise that ethics requires us to risk ourselves precisely at *moments of unknowingness*, when what forms us diverges from what lies before us, when our *willingness to become undone* in relation to others constitutes our chance of becoming human. To be undone by another is a primary necessity, an anguish, to be sure, but also a chance – to be addressed, claimed, bound to what is not me, but also to be moved, to be prompted to act, to address myself elsewhere, and so to vacate the self-sufficient "I" as a kind of possession. If we speak and try to give an account from this place, we will not be irresponsible, or, if we are, we will surely be forgiven.
>
> (Butler 2005, p. 136, my emphasis)

Butler advocates that, 'at moments of unknowingness . . . our willingness to become undone in relation to others constitutes our chance of becoming human'. This refers to those moments when a teacher or learner is confronted by events (or information) that do not correspond to the accepted practices (or ways of knowing) with which she is familiar. In these occasions of 'unknowing', if a trainee or trainer is able to think beyond the 'self-sufficient I', or to take a risk by stepping away from what is familiar and known (i.e. to encounter the unknown), then, from a pedagogic perspective, the outcome can lead to a deeper and more profound understanding. Such may also reconfigure the relation between trainer and trainee in a manner that permits the trainee to be viewed as not deficient or lacking but, rather, knowledgeable in ways that are unappreciated or unacknowledged within the dominant mode of training and practice.

Norms in training are necessary to establish stability and organised structure, so that teachers and learners, alike, get a sense of what must be taught and how this is best accomplished. They are also essential for setting a good standard of practice that ensures the safety and welfare of patients. However, norms are problematic if and when they obscure ways of learning that, while legitimate, lie outside the scope of these norms.

7.8   Power relations that exist in training systems/ relationships: the power of the norm

> We are used to thinking of power as what presses on the subject from outside, as what subordinates, sets underneath, and relegates to a lower order. This is surely a fair description of part of what power does. But if, following Foucault, we understand power as forming the subject as well, as providing the very condition of its existence and the trajectory of desire, then power is not simply what we oppose but also, in a strong sense, what we depend on for our existence and what we harbour and preserve in the beings that we are.
>
> (Butler 1997, pp. 1–2)

In this statement, Butler emphasizes how power exists as an external force that we resist yet also depend upon, to the extent that it is implicated in how we become who we are. Butler extends Michel Foucault's ideas to theorise that, in relations of power, the 'doer' and the 'act' are fused as one and the same thing. In other words, in any situation we tend to act in particular ways that conform, in order to receive recognition.

However, despite these normalising processes, other ways of behaving can also emerge, as in the earlier instance where Mark, newly designated as a trainee, begins to question the wisdom behind his training placement in a speciality he is already an expert in. This illustrates Butler's notion of *performative resignification*, that is, giving new meanings to ways of behaving or acting by questioning the norms that inform action, so that the limits of these norms can be extended to conceive new or different ways of behaving. However, in the context of training, as demonstrated by Mark's story, it can be particularly challenging and difficult to overcome the power of the norm. In querying the deanery's proposal, Mark was challenging at least two norms established by the training body. First, the deanery (i.e. not the trainee) is authorised with the necessary expertise and knowledge to identify the best education and training plans for doctors in training. Second, there exist established boundaries (the norms) that predefine and pre-assess the ways in which a trainee is expected to think and act. That is, the deanery expects Mark to comply with the arrangements made for his training. His actions, then, challenged the authority of the deanery and disrupted the hierarchy of power relations between trainee and training body. Butler would posit that his attempts at resignification (i.e. assigning new meanings to something) were precipitated by an encounter with practice that in some way forced him to question the normative structures.

How events of practice compel surgeons and other practitioners to question or *re-think* the norms that have structured their practice, to date, is a recurring and dominant theme of this book. Resultant and new normative frameworks may emerge from the ways in which clinical environments are organised and structured to deliver services. Examples include restricted waiting times in outpatient clinics, practical activities to reduce infection rates (e.g. the handwashing protocol) or the out-of-hours on-call schedule to provide patient care on the ward. The norms of practice also arise from the attitudes and behaviours that develop as the physician attempts to negotiate the different tensions in her routine practice. All these competing factors can affect how a surgeon responds to unanticipated encounters with patients.

In the penultimate chapter, I closely examine the ideas of practice generated by the impact of these norms on the clinical experience of surgeons.

References

Butler, J. (2005). *Giving an Account of Oneself.* Fordham University Press.

Department of Health. (1995). *Hospital Doctors: Training for the Future.* Working Group on Specialist Medical Training. London: Department of Health.

General Medical Council. (2010). *Final Report of the Education and Training Regulation Policy Review: Recommendations and Options for the Future Regulation of Education and Training.* London: General Medical Council.

Intercollegiate Surgical Curriculum (ISC). (2016). *The Intercollegiate Surgical Curriculum for General Surgery.* Retrieved from www.iscp.ac.uk/curriculum/surgical/spe cialty_year_syllabus.aspx?enc=Ttek+oCN/eOTQZ3fsf5KIg.

Lacan, J. (1993). *Seminar 3: The Psychoses,* trans. Grigg, R. New York: W. W. Norton.

Norcini, J. J. (2003). "Work Based Assessment." *British Medical Journal,* 326: 753–755.

Norcini, J. J. (2007). "Workplace-Based Assessment in Clinical Training." In Swanwick, T. (Ed.), *Understanding Medical Education.* Edinburgh: Association for the Study of Medical Education.

Norcini, J. J., and Burch, V. (2007). "Workplace-Based Assessment as an Educational Tool: AMEE Guide No 31." *Medical Teacher,* 29: 855–871.

Norcini, J. J., Sturmans, F., Drop, R., et al. (2003). "The Mini-CEX: A Method for Assessing Clinical Skills." *Annals of Internal Medicine,* 138: 476–481.

Phillips, A. W., and Jones, A. E. (2015). "The Validity and Reliability of Workplace Based Assessments in Surgical Training." *The Bulletin,* 97 (3): e19–e23.

Porter, R. (1997). *The Greatest Benefit to Mankind.* London: Harper Collins.

Postgraduate Medical Education and Training Board (PMETB). (2005). *Workplace Based Assessment.* Postgraduate Medical Education and Training Board.

(RCPSC) Royal College of Physicians and Surgeons of Canada. (2015). *CanMEDS 2015 Physician Competency Framework.* Retrieved from www.royalcollege.ca/rcsite/docu ments/canmeds/canmeds-full-framework-e.pdf.

Scott, D. (2014). *Gilbert Simondon's Psychic and Collective Individuation: A Critical Introduction and Guide.* Edinburgh: Edinburgh University Press.

Simondon, G. (1989). *Individuation Psychique et Collective.* Paris: Aubier.

Usher, R., and Edwards, R. (1994). *Postmodernism and Education.* London: Routledge.

Zizek, S. (1989). *The Sublime Object of Ideology.* Verso Books.

8 How Does The Structurisation of Medical Practice Enable and Control The Ways in Which Practice is Lived and Realised?

The structurisations of practice refer to the normative frameworks that organise and create the design and delivery of clinical care. These include; the on-call schedule, hospital or clinic waiting times, health policy, the organisation and deployment of hospital services and the outcomes agenda for patient care and clinical training. As such, these 'structures' *affect* the thoughts, emotions and actions that emerge when dealing with unexpected clinical encounters. This chapter examines how these formal structurisations of medical practice control the ways in which surgeons think, problem solve and act: how they *actualise* their practice. The chapter concludes by querying how the affective conditions of practice are expressed in surgeons' attitudes and behaviours.

Accounts of practice from Eleanor and Miranda (two surgeons) provide the setting in which to unpack these concepts. These surgeons discuss, in these excerpts, on-call and emergency work in which they encountered unexpected clinical problems that forced them to rethink their practices.

8.1 Eleanor's story

Eleanor, a final year surgical trainee based in London, describes her training as a 'disappointing experience'. She had gained entry onto a highly competitive specialty training programme (a ratio of 12 candidates to each training place) and expected a defined period of formal training with skilled mentors. Instead, Eleanor opines that the training programme failed to provide necessary opportunities to acquire fundamental technical and practical skills. She identifies a number of factors which collectively diminish the objectives of surgical training: an insufficient volume of operations, a lack of keen and able surgical trainers who prioritise teaching in the operating theatre, the lethargic culture of the NHS and the service pressures brought to bear on it.

> The anaesthetists are slow and discouraged and the theatre staff have low morale and low motivation and the theatre is hideously inefficient and the whole system is against you. Then there is the pressure of targets to get the operation done. So, if there's space for you to be taken through an operation, it's just wiped out routinely. . . . It's becoming evident that trainees are doing absolutely nothing, they are just assisting. Six years of assisting does not make you a surgeon.

Her dejection, anger and exasperation are expressed clearly throughout the interview, as she thoughtfully describes her experiences of training and providing care for patients. The emotions she expresses (as a consequence of her encounters with practice) provide an insight into the affective conditions of everyday clinical work that have influenced and determined her attitudes, behaviour and outlook on professional practice. Her statement articulates the shared opinion of all the surgeons I interviewed, namely, that the working culture and practices of the NHS, including staff attitudes and conduct, make surgical training difficult to initiate and sustain. Eleanor insists that surgical training must involve dedicated supervision and guidance of trainees (by trainers) undertaking operative procedures. Assisting a consultant is not on par with the valuable experience of operating with supervision. She also emphasises that facilitating effective operative training requires greater support from the wider surgical team, as well as from hospital systems and services.

I asked Eleanor if she could remember a clinical experience that transformed her practice by altering her thinking and behaviour. She recalled two clinical events that occurred during her on-call shifts. Before addressing her experiences, it is worth briefly examining the clinical context of her on-call duties, which frames her encounters with practice. During Eleanor's training, her responsibilities as the on-call surgeon included the overnight management of all surgical inpatients. In addition, she was expected to review and treat emergencies (e.g. bleeding from trauma, perforation of the bowel) or urgent surgical problems (e.g. abdominal pain secondary to an inflamed appendix or gallbladder).

However, as is commonplace across emergency departments in the UK, the majority of patients attending A&E do not require emergency care, though they may need investigation of their symptoms, as well as reassurance. But Eleanor's expectation was that she would only be called by staff in the A&E department if there was a dangerously sick patient who needed immediate operative intervention. Anything less than these circumstances should, in her opinion, be managed by the emergency staff. She referenced her previous duties and responsibilities as an A&E doctor to support and validate her views and expectations of how patients in the A&E department should be cared for and by whom.

Eleanor's second account relates to her experience of working long hours as part of a multi-disciplinary team in a specialist cancer centre. Tensions and conflicts can arise between team members, especially when individual workloads are overflowing, leading to disputes on who should assume overall responsibility for specific clinical problems. Eleanor told me that she is frequently expected to 'sort things out', even when the clinical problem does not directly relate to her skill set. She faces this difficulty in this second story when she discusses responsibility for post-surgery pain management.

Pain in the middle of the night

(I have transformative experiences) all the time. . . . That's the only way that I've learnt anything. I was called down to Casualty (A&E) one night and it was when breech times were becoming tight. It was about 3 o'clock in the morning. "Can you come downstairs and see this nine-year old boy who has pain?" I was like, "well, it's 3 o'clock in the morning why has he turned up now with pain?!" I asked the nurse to get one of their A&E doctors to see him and establish what the problem was. I got another doctor ringing back to say I'd really appreciate your opinion about this child's pain. There was a change in culture going on where I felt it was very disrespectful of my time basically and I had previously worked as a junior in A&E where you tried to do the best you could for the patient yourself and when you needed a specialist opinion then you called on a specialist. But I felt that in this case they (the A&E staff) hadn't done the basics . . . not taken a good history of the problem or performed some discriminatory tests.

Anyway, the long and short of it was that I was in a bad mood. I had to get up and go down there and assess the patient and send them home as quick as possible. I went down there and it was a Bengali family and, to make matters worse, the dad started trundling on about housing benefit and how they needed to move house because the kid couldn't walk up and down the stairs properly because he was constantly tired. This is all leading up to the fact that everything was in place for me to make a mistake based on irritating situational factors. Thank the lord I didn't do that! I had a chat with the nine-year-old boy who had non-specific abdominal pain. I took him into a room, pulled his clothes up and noticed a slight fullness on the right side of his abdomen. He had a Wilm's tumour (a form of kidney cancer in children). I spotted that . . . did the necessary investigations etc. and he was sent to a specialist centre to have big cancer surgery aged nine years.

That transformed my practice immediately, because I thought when GPs, or A&E nurses or doctors ring you up, they may or may not know what they're doing, they may not have even done the basics. They may or may not be polite. Whatever. But basically, if they know what they're doing and they've asked you to see the patient, you should see the patient. If they don't know what they're doing and they ask you to see the patient, then you should still see the patient. It transformed my attitude to that . . . it made me a safer doctor. I was having to do a lot more work now, which previously would have been done by other people. But it was a warning to me and thankfully I heeded it.

Post-surgery pain

When I was working in Hopgood, we had a young woman who had a sarcoma (muscle tumour) in her pelvis. Having had a load of chemo and everything. She came back to the ward post surgery and in the morning she was very unwell, dropped her blood pressure, very unwell. I was running around thinking she's picked up an infection after the chemo. I sorted her out, stabilised her. It was a bunker job, where we would get there at 7 in the morning and leave at 9pm. We were leaving the building one evening when one of the nurses said to me, "this epidural is not working," and I asked her to call the anaesthetic team who deal with epidurals.

The next morning I came back to find that the patient had a compartment syndrome (a serious muscle condition that can result in the loss of a limb), masked by the epidural, and had lost part of her leg. When the nurse had told me that the "epidural was not working," she had come to this conclusion because the patient had complained of leg pain. But at the time I didn't know about the leg pain and the nurse had not told me either, possibly because she assumed that I understood that "epidural not working" meant that the patient was experiencing leg pain. Any leg pain post-surgery would immediately mandate a careful medical review.

That (episode) transformed my practice because now if a nurse says anything to me on my way out, I say, "what do you mean?" I take more responsibility now, I ask more questions. If a nurse comes up to you and says something, then it's because they're worried about something. They're questioning you because they're worried. That was a serious error and I'm not going to say it was all my fault, but I was part of a cascade of disastrous events.

I want to focus on three key themes that arise from these narratives of practice. The first concerns the affects and emotions precipitated when negotiating the *structurisations of medical practice*: the ways in which hospital clinical practice is constructed, organised and represented. Second, what is the role of this structurisation of medical practice in both enabling and also controlling the manner in which Eleanor actualises her practice? Put another way, how do the structures and organisation of clinical medicine condition how Eleanor sees, understands and acts within an event of practice? Third, what are the ways in which Eleanor experiences the clinical encounter, and, relatedly, how is she *capacitated* to produce particular ways of thinking, being and doing?

Structurisations of clinical practice include hospital policies such as waiting times, shift systems, hospital-at-night arrangements, staff hierarchy and dynamics and interpersonal relationships between members of different specialty teams all determine how clinical events are affectively experienced and understood. The affective consequences precipitated by these institutional frameworks of clinical practice influence and mould emerging professional identities, with great impact on how individuals form, develop and account for their personal sense of professional responsibility, duty and integrity.

As seen in earlier chapters, formal instructions on conduct and duty (presented in professional handbooks by regulatory authorities) can fall short in instigating the desired changes to behaviours and attitudes. As Eleanor and other surgeons in this book have demonstrated, encountering the uncertainty of practice as it arises, and thus being impelled to engage with the thisness of events, cultivates an understanding of one's professional roles and responsibilities in ways that are meaningful, enduring and ultimately transformative of earlier practice. Henceforth, new ways of thinking and acting emerge in one's own practice. To explore these themes further I borrow from Gilles Deleuze's theory of the actual-virtual.

8.2 How is Eleanor's practice actualised?

In *Difference and Repetition* (1994, Chapter 5), Deleuze discusses how individuals are neither isolated nor discrete entities. Instead, he suggests that individuals are made up of an ongoing series of *relations* that connect the sensations, emotions and thoughts with the intensities that trigger them. These intensities, or affective relations, have the capacity to produce specific outcomes of behaviour or *actualisations* (Smith 2012, 253).

Daniel Smith (2012) articulates Deleuze's view that the way in which something develops is 'objectively problematic' (p. 253), meaning it cannot be predicted ahead of time. Applying this to the case of Eleanor, it is not known exactly how she will act from moment to moment during her on-call shift. This unknown course of action is what Deleuze terms the 'virtual' or 'potential' (Whitehead uses the same term) dimension: thoughts, behaviours etc. which have *not* been previously conceived or experienced, and therefore once actualised are novel ways of being. The virtual (potential) represents what *can* happen: how Eleanor may choose to act and react. This is distinct to *what-is-possible*.

Specifically, Deleuze asserts that the 'possible' refers to what is already known or what has come to pass or exist, that is, *an already-conceptualised outcome*. For example, Eleanor may have chosen to behave in the following ways: refusing to see the patient, reiterating to the emergency team that this patient was their responsibility to manage, asking the patient to return during daytime hours, reviewing the patient but missing the diagnosis because her irritable mood occludes her ability *to be open* to the clinical problem or reviewing the patient but missing the diagnosis because she approaches the clinical problem with fixed ideas of what the cause may be. These forms of responding are established patterns of behaviour and may have been 'acted out' (i.e. actualised) in the past. However, these *possible* ways of behaving do not contribute towards creating new thoughts or behaviours for Eleanor, nor do they expand her capacities beyond what is known. That is the distinction between the 'possible' and the 'virtual/potential'.

Eleanor's actions that night took on a different course for her; she made a choice to persevere with the clinical event, and to be curious and responsive to what initially appeared to be an irritating set of circumstances. She actualised one of the infinite virtualities – the encounter with the child generated new insights into clinical practice that she had neither conceived nor anticipated prior to the event, and which proceeded to alter her approach to surgical practice. She detected a rare childhood tumour by engaging with an unusual problem and in so doing transformed her understanding of what it means to provide surgical care for a patient. Here, new modes of thinking and doing emerged from the relations that formed and developed in the encounter between how she viewed herself, her practice, her colleagues and her patients. In Eleanor's own words, the experience was a 'warning sign' against her complacency in practice. Therefore, the virtual/potential created new relationalities and new connectivities within her practice which, in turn, have helped her become a more careful, more thoughtful and 'safer doctor'.

The second narrative involving Eleanor, in this chapter (see page 139), reveals a very different and almost opposing outcome. But it still brought about a learning event for her. In this encounter, Eleanor takes the routine clinical pathway, follows established clinical procedure and refers the nurse to the pain team. In pursuing this course of action, her behaviours are an example of the *possible* rather than the virtual/potential. After passing on the nurse's request to see the patient on account of the epidural not working, Eleanor learns the grave outcome for the patient the next day. The patient was suffering pain due to a developing surgical pathology, which soon claimed the patient's leg. Eleanor then realises that she should have responded differently to the nurse's request, because it signified a serious concern that the nurse was unable to verbalise appropriately, perhaps due to the relation of authority and power that invariably complicates the relationship between the two healthcare professionals.

This illustrates how one example of the structurisation of medical practice – the hospital hierarchy and its associated power relations – can control Eleanor's actualisation of her duties and, in fact, obscure her immediate understanding of her responsibilities. Eleanor speaks of how this event transformed her, so that now she listens carefully when a nurse poses questions or makes requests, because she realises that such may indicate real clinical concerns. These changes in attitude and behaviour were precipitated once Eleanor was confronted with the consequences to the patient the following day. This event opened up the *virtual* realm for her, identifying for Eleanor how that encounter revealed other ways to act which extended her existing capacities to see and understand in practice.

What factors influence or enable certain thoughts and actions?

An important question arises from both of the above encounters presented by Eleanor, and it concerns the processes of actualisation, that is, how she chose to act in the certain ways that she did. For example, in the first narrative, why did she initially encounter the patient referral as an irritant, how and why did her response to see and treat the child become actualised, and how did a particular solution emerge from the problem? While these questions do touch on issues of clinical decision making, they are more specifically aimed (herein) at querying how we are *enabled to act* in specific ways when immersed in the contingent nature of clinical practice. This is the central theme of this final part of the chapter.

It is difficult to predict or anticipate how clinical events may unfold at any one moment. As medicine is a discipline grounded in science, fact and evidence-based practice, one may expect clinical decision-making to be a transparent process dependent on a rational evaluation of indisputable facts. But the process of *acting on* factual data cannot solely be reduced to a linear sequence of discrete steps. As seen in earlier narratives such as the story of Mr. Pitt's stent insertion (see Chapter 4) as well as in the aforementioned clinical accounts, clinical decision making is steeped in the '*messiness*' of human interactions and relations. In the theoretical chapter (see Chapter 2), I discussed Barad's notion of *intra-actions*, that is, the idea that agency[1] arises from the relations that emerge between human actants (previous experiences, affects, thoughts, bodies) and non-human actants (examination findings, radiological images of a tumour, the on-call pager, discourses on patient care, concepts of ethics). In adhering to this model, then, we cannot anticipate Eleanor's process of clinical decision-making or its outcome. That is, both these elements are contingent on a series of intra-actions that form and develop within the clinical encounter, and which therefore cannot be predicted in advance of the event of practice. How Eleanor takes account of or *prehends* (Whitehead 1929, p. x) all the elements that constitute the encounter is linked to how her practice matters to her, and this cannot be known in advance. Such adds, then, another layer of complexity to an already mysterious process. The formation of these prehensive relations is distinct from concepts of cause and effect, and also from subject-object dichotomies.

8.3   How does the structurisation of medical practice impact emotional states?

In the first narrative, Eleanor is aware of her emotive state ('I was in a bad mood'), even identifying the triggers for it: an unsatisfactory encounter with emergency department staff on the phone, a perception of disappointing workplace etiquette, a sense of being disrespected, unmet expectations of colleagues and annoyance at the patient's father's comments. States of emotion reflect the continuous flow of affect, which suffuses every encounter with practice, and which constructs and (in)forms one's thoughts, feelings and actions. Eleanor is very aware of the effect of these emotional tensions, remarking that, 'everything was in place for me to make a mistake based on irritating situational factors'. She opines that the culmination of these triggers had proceeded to structure the encounter in such a way that circumstances were ripe for a potential serious error of practice (and subsequent disastrous outcome).

Eleanor argued with emergency staff because she viewed the patient referral as inappropriate, exemplifying how actualisations of practice in the out-of-hours service (e.g. tensions between colleagues and arguments regarding clinical responsibility of the patient) are influenced and controlled by hospital working practices and culture. Later, she describes the expectations made of her, such expectations having been created by the way in which patient care at night is organised: 'I had to get up and go down there (to A&E) and assess the patient and send them home as quick as possible'.

The way in which Eleanor both becomes a subject of this framework of practice, and also identifies herself within its boundaries, is an example of an interpellation, a process first discussed in length by Louis Althusser (1971). Interpellation, put simply, refers to the notion that ideas we form are not a product of our own thought processes but are rather the result of the ideologies we imbibe, albeit unknowingly. For example, we are surrounded by (and frequently encounter) external ideas on all aspects of life such as culture, gender, class and race. Such ideas are presented in ways that cause us to internalize and accept them as our own. For example, from the point of birth, we are interpellated into assigned gender roles, evidenced by our collective, societal tendency to dress girls in pink and boys in blue.

Similarly, the structurisations of medical practice – the A&E waiting times and the penalties for breeching them, the limited access to radiological investigations, the reduced staff presence at night – interpellate Eleanor as a particular kind of medical subject. In the first narrative, Eleanor is a clinician tasked with managing surgical emergencies and specific, pre-identified surgical problems, deciding quickly if patients need to be admitted or discharged home. However, the young boy who came to A&E was not a surgical emergency, though his cancer diagnosis needed urgent attention. Processes of interpellation have two important effects. First, they contribute to the affective responses that emerge from practice. Second, they can obscure and occlude a surgeon's capacity to access the virtual dimension of their practice (i.e. to think and act in ways that create new modes of understanding and behaving in practice).

In my individual practice as a teacher and trainer, I ask my experienced trainees to think about how they can 'shake off' the shackles that arise from what they have read, been taught or believe to be their professional responsibilities. It represents an effort to encourage learners to attempt to exceed their clinical duties and limits of practice, and to seek a more personal and enduring understanding of what they can become as surgeons and practitioners. To do this is to be wholly capacitated within an encounter in ways that allow one to answer the question posed by Baruch Spinoza and others, namely, 'What *can* I do in this situation' rather than 'what *must* I do in these circumstances?' I expand on these ideas later in the chapter, when I explore the notion of practical ethics.

8.4   'Thinking feeling': affect can mediate how we come to know the world

The pedagogical task of surgical educators is to consider how one attempts to capture the ways in which the clinical event resonates with the learner (i.e. the internal resonance of the event of practice), because this addresses what matters for the trainee in a learning encounter. What are the different ways in which the trainee engages with the clinical encounter?

Deleuze proposes that experiencing within an encounter can spark powerful affective forces, or a *series of intensities*, that arise from the relationalities (i.e. how one relates to something) that develop. These relations are not static events between subject-subject or subject-object. Rather, affective relations refer to dynamic, local intensities of affect that form and develop within the flows of any experience. Through affect, an individual grasps the experience, or, the thisness, of the encounter, reflecting how that event matters to her. For example, Eleanor's bad mood is an emotive state created by the series of affects that emerge from her on-call encounter with the young boy in pain, and these intensities constitute her experience of that event of practice.

Affect is both precognitive and pre-linguistic, arising before the emergence of familiar or recognisable emotions that could provide a context to the experience.

For these reasons, Gilbert Simondon (Mills 2016) has suggested that affect provides a structure or form to the substance of the encounter. When immersed in the uncertainty of an unfolding event, the development of affective relations within that experience allows the individual to grasp something as she struggles to make sense of the substance of the unknown encounter, attempts to find meaning in the experience and decides upon how to act appropriately.

Eleanor engages with the encounter initially through such intensities. These intensities constitute the initial form of her experience and reflect how the encounter matters to her. By 'mattering', I refer back to the notion of prehension (Whitehead 1929), that is, how she takes account of things within the encounter, how she affects the relations and how, in turn, she is affected in the relations. In this example, Eleanor experiences the encounter with the child, the encounter with a slightly abnormal looking abdomen, the encounter with her own expectations of colleagues, the encounter with the radiological images of the child's abdomen, the encounter with her prejudices regarding social housing and welfare and the encounter with herself as a practitioner who is safer and more responsible now. The ways in which she prehends affect certain intensities that subsequently activate her to think and act in particular ways. Through this Simondonian conception of experience and encounter, the individual is transformed from a 'being' to an 'act' (Barthelemy 2015, p. 26).

8.5　Miranda's story

Miranda is a consultant surgeon and senior lecturer of five years standing. She works in a central London teaching hospital. She completed the majority of her surgical training in hospitals within London and Essex. She had a strong interest in clinical research as a trainee and undertook a research degree as part of her training. Her present role is split between NHS clinical work and academic research. However, she is frustrated by the increasing demands of her surgical practice, which encroach on time that she feels should be spent conducting research and supervising PhD students. She is exasperated by the fragmentation of her junior surgical team.

> Well I think the first thing to say is that there is nobody to train! My clinics . . . I don't have a registrar, be it for training or service and I have set up the clinics in a way which means I don't need them (the trainees) because it's too unreliable to rely on their presence. Initially, when they were available it was not reliable to depend on them because they would be away doing nights or whatever, so you can't run a service this way . . . Theatre lists . . . you do have somebody to train, but usually . . . the person who's in theatre on Wednesday is often off after an on-call night, so I end up texting them to give them a heads up, which other (consultants) don't do, and you can complain about the trainees but at the end of the day it's the system.
>
> 　Emergencies . . . I am increasingly called to go and just deal with I (there is no junior trainee who goes ahead and reports back). So, as a trainer, well,

there is nobody to train! And also it's very difficult to train because you don't know what their training needs are because you're not seeing them on a regular basis.

Miranda's anxieties and complaints about the way in which the hospital and clinical schedule is organised ('the system') are common threads found in all the interviews conducted for this book. There is an exasperation that both the shift system and the organisation of the hospital prevent the existence of teams of surgeons who work and train together consistently, which could build an enhanced system of education and training, establish a happy work camaraderie and define both shared responsibilities and common goals.

Similar to Eleanor's story, here, the hospital structures and working patterns (i.e. structurisations of practice) control actualisations of practice. For example, Miranda describes her aggravation at the lack of a trainee presence during her weekly Wednesday operating list. The hospital is legally required to ensure that the trainees who have worked overnight are sent home to rest. However, some trainees, mindful that they are missing out on valuable opportunities to operate, practice and learn, attend the operating list anyway. Miranda looks upon these trainees kindly and will often alert them via text message regarding which surgical cases are scheduled and who the patients are. However, the surgical tradition is such that, in order to attend an operating list and be taught, trainees are expected to come into work early on that morning (i.e. usually by 7am), to see all the pre-operative patients, to read the notes on those patients, to be familiar with the relevant medical information and to prepare patients for surgery. This is especially challenging to achieve for a trainee who has been on-call the previous night and subsequently busy organising an appropriate patient handover.

For Miranda, the structurisations of hospital practice control the way in which she actualises her surgical practice. An example is how she organises her clinic to function without trainee involvement.

In this narrative, Miranda describes her early experiences of dealing with ruptured aortic aneurysms, encounters that transformed her practice and attitude toward patient care. For context, an aneurysm is an abnormal dilatation of the main blood vessel in the body (aorta), which places it at risk of rupture. Such ruptures are frequently fatal. In some situations, it is not possible to provide any life-saving interventions, and patients are treated palliatively.

When there is no operative solution

Everybody thinks that a (aneurysm) rupture is so exciting and you want to do the surgery. But then there are the cases you can't operate on because it's too late. What I hadn't realized back then was that sometimes patients with a ruptured aneurysm (who are unsuitable for surgery) don't die that quickly, so you put them in a side-room. But they're still alive the next day, what do you do then? You've already told the family and relatives the night before that the prognosis is very poor. And now that they are relatively stable, well, can they go home? Can they die at home?

I remember that the first time that became difficult for me was somebody who was still stable about 24 hours later, quite comfortable and the family said we would like to take her home, so we put her in an ambulance and then she became unstable so she came back to us and died in the hospital. And that was obviously traumatic for everyone. . . . Nowadays, people expect the full explanation, they normally will understand but then it's when the patient doesn't die . . . (the family will say)"are you sure?" . . . Even though we have a CT confirmed diagnosis. We get asked, "will they be aware? Will they slip away?" Sometimes they do, sometimes they don't. . . .

Recently on an on-call I found that I wanted to spend more time with that patient and their family than someone we would take to theatre and operate on. Because I think, if you're explaining an operation to a patient, the family, they understand and they have questions, you explain and get on with it. But in this sort of situation (where there's no life-saving procedure available), you can imagine it's very difficult (for the patient and family) to understand. . . . Very often it's too tempting for the team to say . . . "the patient is still alive, we'll address all the symptoms, make sure they're not in pain." And then it's very tempting to say, "there are no more decisions to be made about this patient" or "we'll see this patient last on the ward round if at all" or "the Palliative team will see them." But actually, that's the family/patient who has the most questions, isn't it? Or another family member will arrive and say, "they're still with us, but for how long?" All those questions I think you cannot give a clear answer to but making a stab at it is important. Whereas, there are other life-threatening conditions where you know you can do an operation and fix it.

(Miranda, consultant surgeon)

The mortality associated with emergency aneurysm surgery is very high. From a purely technical stance, the steps of an aneurysm surgery involve making big incisions, dissecting a considerable amount of tissue, controlling rapid and catastrophic bleeding and doing all of this whilst aware of the fact that the patient may die on the operating table. The surgeon needs to be decisive, quick and fluent in their technique. The heroic, intra-operative efforts can appear exciting for a trainee who is enthused and keen to learn surgical method.

Miranda was initially excited at the prospect of participating in aneurysm surgery. However, she had not expected to be the most *affected* by those patients for whom she could never provide an operative solution. In this scenario, the actualisation of the virtual occurs for her when confronted by the patient who is still alive following a ruptured aneurysm. She is affectively capacitated in this moment before being able to *think through* why she feels this way. Massumi describes what occurs in these initial affective moments:

You own the feeling as your own, and recognise it as a content of your life, an episode in your personal history. But in the instance of the *affective hit*, there is no content yet. All there is is the affective quality, coinciding with the feeling of the interruption. . . . That affective quality is all there is to the world in that instant. It takes over life, fills the world, for an immeasurable instant of shock.

(2008, p. 5, my emphasis)

The 'affective hit' in Miranda's account exists as the intensities precipitated when she sees that her patient is still alive and yet to die, the following day. The expressions of affect may be imperceptible, sometimes manifesting as a stunned silence, the individual standing agape, a quickening of the heartbeat or teary eyes. The intensities have not been explicated or interpreted into rational thought or meaningful emotion: 'there is no content yet.' For example, no emotion of sadness or anger has evolved in the moment of the affective hit. Her *feelings* (Whitehead 1929) or affective intensities rupture 'the world' of surgery and human life as she has come to know and understand it. The encountered concept of patient-still-alive-and-yet-to-die does not fit into the transcendent categories that she has read about in textbooks or been advised on by her community of mentors and peers. Namely, this patient does not neatly fit into the 'survived the rupture' or 'died from the rupture' categories. The latter and former outcomes belong to the realm of the *possible*: consequences that are known about and have come to pass.

For Miranda, the affective interruptions of this encounter are precognitive and prelinguistic, asserting the effect of Alain Badiou's (2001) 'event' (first discussed in Chapter 1). Her pre-existing understanding and knowledge of aneurysm pathology, surgical intervention and the human condition are *punctured* by the reality of a yet-to-die patient: 'the event . . . compels the subject to invent a new way of being and acting in the situation' (Badiou 2001, p. 42). Miranda's 'new way of being and acting' translated into a desire to spend more time with the families of patients she is not able to operate on. She rationalises after the affective hit that it makes sense to do so, because these families have the most questions (owing to the confusing but fatal outcome). In these experiences of affect, Miranda is activated to think and behave in ways that are not just compassionate but that also demonstrate a new understanding of the nuances and complexities of the human condition.

Massumi iterates that the ability to affect and, in turn, be affected causes a transition between 'one state of capacitation to a *diminished* or *augmented* state of capacitation' (2008, p. 2). In other words, the affective experience can equally precipitate an enhanced level of thought and action, as well as a 'diminished' approach. For example, Miranda observes that patients close to death may not require any active clinical intervention (e.g. medication or a blood transfusion), and this can lead to doctors removing themselves from any direct involvement with the patient or family. I suggest that these attitudes and behaviours in practice are akin to a diminishment in one's capacity to act in ways that exceed conventional approaches. However, Miranda's affective encounters with a morbid clinical experience have enabled her to view the situation differently. For example, her process of affectation has compelled her to attempt answering difficult questions posed by patients (in similar situations) and their families.

The discussion extends naturally, now, to the question of how and why some surgeons or clinicians would behave differently in the same circumstances. Included in this is this question: can affect diminish across time, as part of a natural process, or, does (and can) an individual choose to alter their experience with affect?

8.6 The pedagogic implications of ruptures in practice

Eleanor and Miranda narrate clinical experiences describing how they reacted and coped with the immediacy of unexpected surgical events that questioned their perception and understanding of practice. Such vignettes portray *disturbances* of practice wherein each surgeon is forced to think and act in ways that were not conceived of prior to the event. I suggest that the interruption to practice shifts the focus from *being* a trainee to *becoming* a surgeon, specifically, from being instructed on what to do and how to think to engaging with difficult emotions and challenging practice.

This engagement has implications for how an individual starts to conceive and develop their sense of what it means to be a professional, and how to act in the best interests of one's patients. First, and more specifically, an individual surgeon constructs her own identifications within her practice, namely, a prioritisation of matters of particular importance to her. Next, a surgeon is allowed a process of becoming, that is, a professional evolution that is unique to herself and her own development of skill and reflection. Finally, the surgeon absorbs an understanding of clinical ethics in an organic manner, through her own experiences of practice, a process by which such ethics become more firmly ingrained than by way of objectively reading about the subject. We now look at each of these implications, in turn.

Surgeon identifications

The narrative accounts demonstrate how *individual identifications* as surgical professionals emerge through experiences with contingent clinical practice. In other words, each surgeon identifies specific priorities that are of concern in surgical practice and which can be traced back to how the clinical encounter mattered to them. For example, Miranda explains that her technical practice will never become stale for her even though she is engaged in repetitive surgeries. Each operative encounter, she believes, affords an opportunity to better the patient experience or improve the team dynamic.

Eleanor, meanwhile, describes herself as a 'safer doctor', who assumes 'more responsibility' after the encounters with patients in pain. The particular priorities voiced by each of these individual surgeons appear to arise as a consequence of how the surgeon engages with or *prehends* the initial clinical event. I suggest that what is occurring in these stories is an account of how that particular individual encounters the *form* of the event of practice, that is, how they grasp the particular clinical event so that it becomes a matter of concern. Thus, the individual sub-jectivities of the two surgeons arise through unique processes of mattering (i.e. how the events of practice are perceived or encountered by Miranda and Eleanor respectively).

For Whitehead (and Deleuze), the individual emerges through the relations she forms within the process of experiencing something, before dissolving in the process of becoming, so that new relations may emerge. For example, Eleanor becomes a subject (comes into being) through the affective relations that arise as she engages in the encounter. Specifically, she affects the encounter (e.g. argues with A&E staff because she feels that her time and specialist skills are not respected, detects something upon examining the young patient which heightens her clinical suspicions) and is, in turn, affected by the encounter (e.g. irritation at being called to see a patient in the early hours, rethinking her practice in light of how a serious and life-altering diagnosis for the patient initially presented as a non-urgent and puzzling referral in the middle of the night). The intensities trig-gered by the immanence of the affective relations cause her to emerge relationally activated and capacitated to think and act in particular ways that were not con-ceived prior to the encounter, but which reflect how the encounter *matters* to her.

The distinction I wish to make here is that official documentations like *GMP* (2013) and *GSP* (2014) interpellate subjects according to prior established and instructive ways of thinking and doing. In reality, a pre-existing surgeon identity does not actually exist; the surgeon emerges through ideological interpellation. Put simply, the inherent capacities that both Miranda and Eleanor possess, namely to act and think in unfamiliar encounters, are not legitimised outside of the documen-tation. Rather, the training materials anticipate a particular surgeon identity, distin-guished by specific and demonstrable skills that are without real clinical context.

What these authorised documents do not recognise or embrace are the affective experiences that suffuse the actual events in which these skills are put into prac-tice. The documents present clinical practice in idealized forms, that is, a sanitary environment devoid of the challenges or conflicting tensions of the real world. In order to encourage the desired clinical behaviours and thereby propagate satisfac-tory patient experiences, there is a requirement to understand the implications of the affective dimensions of practice.

Immanent practice emphasises a process of becoming

The individuation of Eleanor and Miranda, through their accounts of practice, illustrates processes of self-transformation in their beliefs and practice. The immanence of each learner's pathway is a story of her becoming, through learn-ing encounters that precipitate new ways of thinking and being.

Norms are individuated

Established criteria of practice interpellate the surgeon as a particular subject of ideological practices and surgical training, because her actions can only be recog-nised and legitimised within that specific framework. However, this is to deny the ability of an individual to individuate through processes of immanent reflection, reflexive practice and critical thought. Through such individuation, the generic medical guidance on practice is transformed in ways that are relevant and meaningful to trainees, as individuals engaged in real practice.

8.5   A clinical ethics based on responding to the singularity of situations

Concerning how care is performed, or thought to be performed, by the doctor, if one were to contrast the deployment of care in the official guidance (GMP 2013; GSP 2014) with the earlier narrative accounts of doctor-patient relations, one will find that two types of ethical codes emerge. First is an ethics predominantly conceived in the medical literature, that is, one underpinned by a moral code and a set of rules and criteria by which to evaluate the thoughts, intentions and behaviours of a physician. Deleuze (Colebrook 2002) stipulates that an ethical code based on morality is founded on a transcendent framework of values, which society or an organisation deem to be important in directing and influencing our thoughts and actions at that moment in time.

The second type is an *ethics of practice*, which emerges from *real events of clinical practice*, wherein the doctor has to make decisions in the 'here and now' according to the contingencies of the actual doctor-patient relations. Deleuze advocates the following conception of ethics: a set of facultative rules that 'evaluate what we do according to the immanent mode of existence that it implies' (Smith 2012, p. 176). Such indicates that, despite criticism to the contrary, Deleuze is not promoting an unethical practice, or practices that are wrong or inappropriate, because there would be no norms by which to judge or assess conduct. Deleuze, for his part, addresses this concern by reiterating that an immanent mode of existence refers to how far we push the limits of what we can achieve in a situation, and well as to what separates us from acting in a certain way. In other words, Deleuze poses the question that an ethics of practice must raise, namely, 'What *can* I do, or, what am I *capable* of doing?' rather than 'What *must* I do?' (which refers to issues of morality).

This is exemplified in Eleanor's second narrative. She is aware of both her clinical duty and ethical responsibility to the adult female patient. However, it is late in the evening, and she is being constantly interrupted by nurses who are making demands she views as inappropriate. In her opinion, there are other members of the team who should first review the patient. She is fatigued and also excited to go home early for a change. These tensions in practice are implicated in her decision making.

A Deleuzian conception of ethics would pose the following questions to direct Eleanor's conduct in an actual event of practice: 'given my power to act, what am I capable of achieving in this situation?', 'what are my capacities of doing?', 'how can I come into active possession of my power?' and 'how can I go to the limit of what I can do?' (derived from Smith 2012, p. 176). In short, Deleuze promotes a view of ethics that is a form of responding to the situation that we, as individuals, find ourselves immersed in. It is characterised by the individual's attempts to consistently push themselves to the limits of what they are capable of 'doing' in that encounter.

Deleuze is critical, meanwhile, of those elements that distance the individual from their inherent power to act. Transcendent frameworks of ethical behaviour may constitute a separation from our power to act. Such frameworks prescribe a fixed response to a situation and thus prevent the individual from 'dreaming' or conceiving other ways to think and act that exceed what is known.

> Rather than judging actions and thoughts by appealing to transcendent or universal values, one evaluates them by determining the mode of existence that serves as their principle. A pluralist method of explanation by immanent modes of existences in this way is made to replace the recourse to transcendent values; an immanent ethical difference.
>
> (Smith 2012, p. 147)

Therefore, ethics (for Deleuze) is not grounded in the notion of the transcendent subject, such as the projected figure of the 'good doctor' in *GMP* (2013), whose actions are recognised within an idealized framework of 'moral practice' but which are not grounded in the realities of clinical medicine (e.g. time constraints, overbooked clinics and staff shortages).

None of this discussion should indicate an advocating, on my part, for a lowering of standards of care. Rather, it is meant to draw attention to how the thisness of practice is a strong factor in influencing and moulding our thoughts and actions, both in ways that can exceed conventional practices as well as fall short of minimum standards.

In the theoretical chapters I made reference to Dennis Atkinson's (2018) example of a waterfall to illustrate affective experiences. I return to that same example once again to conclude the earlier remarks. Atkinson compares the unique, dual experiences of standing inside a waterfall (and the states of affect that emerge from within) and standing outside on the banks of a river, observing the waterfall at a distance. When one is caught in the strong rushes of water, whilst standing within the waterfall, one can experience powerful affective states that are triggered by the force of the flows of water. For example, the crashing flows of water may leave you utterly terrified or supremely exhilarated. This lies in stark contrast to the affect precipitated by the act of watching the same process unfold from a distance, on the riverbanks. One may still feel a sense of thrill or fear, but the experience is more local and intense for the individual standing within. For the purposes of the present discussion, this standing within the waterfall represents the immanent nature of experience, capturing the flows of affect and emotion. This is a useful analogy when thinking about how we experience something in the moment, as contrasted with how we experience it later when recalling, recollecting or reflecting on something. The latter is also how teachers observe or assess a trainee, but, in this manner, they cannot know how the trainee experiences or feels encounters with practice.

How is a mode of existence determined? The learner (or teacher) arises out of a specific instance of learning (or teaching), rather than through the assessment criteria of a WBA, for example. The subject, as such, does not exist prior to the experience. The mode of being is determined either through the power to act in an encounter, and by the relations of affectivity, or through the inability of the subject to act to their fullest capacity. Therefore, Deleuze moves beyond a process of judgement facilitated by reference to norms. Instead, he advocates that individuals should look to see whether their actions are in keeping with their full capacity to act in a given situation. Through an augmented state of capacitation, the individual brings about a self-transformation and the potential to create new modes of existence.

To prioritise a notion of immanence in teaching and learning is to subscribe to an ethics of immanence wherein the pedagogical priority is to try to understand learning from the perspective of the learner's capacities to grow. This does not include judgment or assessment of such capacities from external criteria. This is not to diminish the need for course materials, syllabi, assessments and the like, all of which help to educate learners in terms of what they need to know (and what skills they need at attain) to manage other human lives. But a pedagogy of immanent ethics goes further, referring to how a teacher may come to better understand the experience of their learner and to assist the learner in unpacking an encounter.

An example of this is the encounter between Eleanor and the child. What caused her to go and meet with the child, and to examine the child as thoroughly as she did, given all the factors that were dissuading her from that particular actualisation of practice? How did the encounter affect her as it did? How did the affective relations emerge to make this a matter of concern for her? These affective relations constitute the immanent criteria that determine how an individual grasps the encounter, that is, what Atkinson (2016) calls a 'necessary transcendence'. Transcendence, as I use the term (following Deleuze), implies appraisal in accordance to some law, body of knowledge or religion, such that what is being considered is assessed using an established way of seeing, practicing, etc. Recall that the notion of immanence relates to that which emerges from within practice, itself. However, that which emerges from within practice may, for the practitioner, be equivalent to a 'necessary transcendence' that allows grasping the meaning of the particular experience of practice.

Therefore, there is a difference between *external transcendence* (with established rules, criteria and methodologies) and *necessary transcendence*, which emerges from within practice and which is constituted by ways of coping with and understanding the flow of practice. This latter form of transcendence encourages a climate of learning (and also of clinical practice) wherein the learner (e.g. surgeon) is sensitive to the nature by which a patient presents with a problem, and subsequently addresses them with a step-by-step approach, as new issues arise. She poses questions, rather than working from universal values that totalise the experience. She decides the path ahead. This is the power of becoming, namely, answering the event and generating the that-which-is-not-yet that, by its nature, exceeds established practices and has the potential to create new worlds of practice. Whitehead (1929), in his theory of experience, places aesthetics before ontology, because he wants to emphasise that 'how' we experience is the primary concern and should be considered before looking at the processes of becoming.

8.6 Final thoughts

The tales of surgical training that unfold in these pages, along with the analysis of educational materials past and present, precipitates a call for emancipation, specifically, a deliverance from entrenched bureaucratic systems of continuous surveillance, relentless assessment, pernicious regulation and a socio-political mantra of tireless reform. It is not contested that these elements of the modern-day surgical education model were well-intentioned, or that they were conceived and designed to primarily protect and promote the welfare and safety of patients (DOH 2000, 2010; NPSA 2009; Berwick 2013; HEE 2016).

However, as the narratives illustrate, the affectations, thoughts and behaviours of the surgeon are dynamic, unanticipated and *affected* by various factors: rotas, schedules, physical fatigue and mood, colleague relationships, policies, preju-dices, bureaucratic inertia and more. Thus, they can neither be accurately pre-dicted nor fully accounted for. Rather, they have to be negotiated or, to use a Simondonian term, *integrated* (Chabot 2003) if the principles of 'good practice' are to prevail.

The difficulty arises when normative criteria, specified by the current system of assessment and evaluation, act to occlude the intensities and ideas precipitated through local flows of experience. The generation of such intensities and ideas is crucial to both learning and constructing meaning out of one's practice. Of course, there is a need to recognise the governance of established and valued procedures in medical practice, which have accumulated and been formalized, across time. But there is also a parallel and equally valid requirement, namely, to acknowledge personal forms of governance-in-practice that emerge from a surgeon's affective grasp of encounters with complex practice.

Note

1 Within philosophy, human agency in simple terms refers to the capacity of human beings to make choices and enact them on the world.

References

Althusser, L. (1971). "Ideology and Ideological State Apparatuses." In *Lenin and Philoso-phy, and Other Essays*, trans. Brewster, B. (pp. 127–188). London: New Left Books.
Atkinson, D. (2018). *Art, Disobedience and Ethics: The Adventure of Pedagogy*. Palgrave Macmillan.
Badiou, A. (2001). *Ethics: An Essay on the Understanding of Evil*. London: Verso.
Barthelemy, J. H. (2015). *Life and Technology: An Inquiry into and Beyond Simondon*. Meson Press EG.

Berwick, D. (2013). *A Promise to Learn – A Commitment to Act*. Retrieved from www.gov.uk/government/uploads/system/uploads/attachment_data/le/226703/Berwick_Report.pdf.

Colebrook, C. (2002). *Gilles Deleuze*. London and New York: Routledge.

Chabot, P. (2003). *The Philosophy of Simondon*, trans. Krefetz, A., and Kirkpatrick, G. Bloomsbury Academic.

Department of Health. (2000). *The NHS Plan: A Plan for Investment, A Plan for Reform*. Retrieved from http://webarchive.nationalarchives.gov.uk/20130107105354/www.dh.gov.uk/prod_consum_dh/groups/dh_digitalassets/@dh/@en/@ps/documents/digitalasset/dh_118522.pdf.

Department of Health. (2010). *Equity and Excellence: Liberating the NHS*. Retrieved from www.gov.uk/government/uploads/system/uploads/attachment_data/file/213823/dh_117794.pdf.

General Medical Council. (2013). *Good Medical Practice*. London: General Medical Council.

Health Education England. (2016). *Improving Safety Through Education and Training*. Retrieved from www.hee.nhs.uk/sites/default/files/documents/FULL%20report%20medium%20res%20for%20web.pdf.

Massumi, B. (2008). "The Thinking-Feeling of What Happens." *A Semblance of a Conversation*. Retrieved from http://inflexions.org/n1_The-Thinking-Feeling-of-What-Happens-by-Brian-Massumi.pdf.

Mills, S. (2016). *Gilbert Simondon: Information, Technology and Media*. London and New York: Rowman & Littlefield.

NHS National Patient Safety Agency (NPSA). (2009). *Saying Sorry When Things Go Wrong, Being Open, Communicating Patient Safety Incidents with Patients, Their Families and Careers*. Retrieved from www.nrls.npsa.nhs.uk/beingopen/.

Royal College of Surgeons of England. (2014). *Good Surgical Practice*. RCSE: Professional Standards.

Smith, D. W. (2012). *Essays on Deleuze*. Edinburgh University Press.

Whitehead, A. N. (1929). *Process and Reality*. New York: The Free Press.

Part IV

Encountering the Reality of Clinical Practice

coping and learning in contingent environments

9 Making Sense of 'Messy' Practice

affective dispositions, the obligations of practice and processes of mattering

Seeing Red

It is 3.37am. Operating theatre 14. Mr. Cunningham, the recipient of the shiny new liver transplant, lies on the operating table, his abdomen sliced open. On the prep table behind me sits a blue tub which holds his shiny new liver, bathed in special juices, glistening under the theatre lights. I pack the insides of his belly with pristine, crisp white swabs – the whites of which instantly disappear, drenched in a deep crimson hue. I glance at the rising tide of blood in the upper cavity of the abdomen: a concave hollow, occupied until a few minutes ago, by a cirrhotic liver – ugly, rotting, bulbous flesh. My hands move quickly and methodically across the four corners of the abdomen. Removing blood-soaked swabs, squeezing out a shower of sticky, scarlet juice that sloshes around in a bucket while the cell saver hoovers up each precious red cell and pumps it back into the patient. The operating theatre is littered with empty bags of various blood products. All given in what is fast becoming a futile attempt to stem catastrophic bleeding.

I say nothing, I am speechless. Speech-less, mute. My feet squelch inside my clogs, a mixture of my sweat and fluid draining from the sides of the operating table. I keep going – this is not what I'm here to do, I think, increasingly angry and irritated. I didn't come here to watch this man exsanguinate to oblivion! And yet, here I am.

EJ, the consultant surgeon in this surgery is annoyed and exasperated. "We have to do better Arundi, really we do. This is not going to work out for him (the patient). . . . Can someone get me Eva on the phone? I want to know why we decided on *this man* for *this transplant*?! Has he got family outside? Who brought him in to hospital? This is really . . . just not good enough! . . ."

I've noticed that the conversation at these moments always takes on the same tone, the same exasperation, the same questions, the same need to blame someone, anyone, when things don't go according to plan. When patients don't return from the operating theatre, leave alone make if off the operating table. In such moments, there is a tendency for surgeons to believe that we can somehow pinpoint a patient's demise to one particular decision. One

wrong move in what is otherwise presented as a flawless game of chess, careful calculation and evaluation gets the patient from waiting list to the operating theatre. The worlds of the operating theatre –excitement, good things,
heroics and success – transforms in minutes or hours to a place of failure,
despair and death. Many worlds inhabit one space, yet I struggle to figure out
just where I should tread, where I should belong.

I glance up at the clock, 3.53am. Someone is holding a mobile phone to
EJ's ear, as he mutters and paces. He walks away from the operating table.
Perhaps he's calling another colleague for help. Perhaps he's arguing with
night staff working at the depleted blood bank, demanding more products
to be sent. Or, perhaps he's scolding the beleaguered Eva. I don't know and
I don't care. I return to Mr. Cunningham's belly which still weeps red. I continue to 'pack and squeeze'.

(Excerpt taken from my surgical journal,
10 August 2011.)

9.1   Moments of rupture: connecting with the intensities and potentials of the learner experience

Mr. Cunningham was pronounced deceased at 4.58am. EJ had vanished from the
operating theatre – later I heard that he had been seen sitting quietly in the men's
changing room, staring at the cracks in the walls. When he emerged just prior
to the morning ward round, he looked exhausted, shoulders slumped and head
stooped. He paused briefly to squeeze my left shoulder and mumbled, 'we just
have to do better, we really must . . . that's all . . .' I spent the next hour methodically sewing up the great gash down the front of Mr. Cunningham's body, looping
large thick suture material through the swollen skin and tissues, washing and preparing his body – disappearing any trace that hinted at the violence of our failed
and frenzied attempts to keep him alive, so that his family would at least be spared
that unthinkable torment.

The extraordinary experiences of living through such encounters with practice,
which are powerful because of the affective rush they elicit and the states of rupture they create can occur in any training environment. These are the moments of
realisation where real learning occurs (Atkinson 2011) – 'what learning can be
beyond the parameters of reproduction, packaged knowledge, traditional skills
and the pragmatic and predictable application of knowledge' (p. 5–6). It is difficult for me to list what I learned that night or quantify what skills I acquired
or even detail how my skill set or notions of professionalism were enhanced or
diminished through the encounter. I could talk about how that moment caused me
to see my revered surgical trainers in a different light, that I learned how to struggle and fight the unstoppable march of death or that aspects of my surgical technique just seemed to 'click' for me afterwards and my overall technique improved
dramatically. But, instead, I would argue that to do so misses the point.

This book argues that these events, these moments of rupture, are critical to
learning. The challenge for the surgical trainer when responding to the 'evental'

experiences of a surgeon in training is to work with the thisness of the situation for the surgeon-in-training. That is, to develop a pedagogy that is grounded in the haecceities of practice, which allows a learner to persevere with the consequences of the event as they arise.

In everyday pedagogical scenarios in an operating theatre, how does a surgeon educator negotiate, as in this example, the thisness of an episode of catastrophic bleeding which may constitute an 'event' (Badiou 2005) for some surgeons-in-training? There is the immediate clinical emergency that must be dealt with absolutely, yet at the same time, one should not lose sight of how this event will unfurl unknown trajectories for the learner. The event may disrupt the ontological state of the learner in ways that are not explicated by established clinical knowledge or the teacher's experience of an exemplar scenario.

The primary challenge for a trainer is to recognise an event, *as perceived by the learner* and to then know how to support and facilitate it so that the learner commits to the truth of the event and can emerge from it with heightened capacities to understand and perform. This is not easy given that the trainer is also immersed in the emergent event of practice with responsibilities for the patient as well as the learner. However, developing an awareness and sensitivity to these pedagogic priorities is a good starting point from which to identify and contemplate *how something becomes an event* for a trainee, and what is needed to support, facilitate and unpack these critical learning encounters in practice.

When encouraging learners to reflect on the episode of practice, it is imperative that the exercise is not only reduced to identifying perceived positive and negative behaviours: 'what did I do well? What could I do better?' If the pedagogic objective is to enhance a learner's ability to function effectively when confronted with the contingency of practice, then I suggest it requires an approach that recognises that how a learner encounters the immanence of an event is intimately connected to how that learner engages with practice in ways that are meaningful to her and which represent how this learning encounter matters to her.

9.2   Suggested principles to guide the development of future pedagogic strategies

The development of pedagogies of encounter identified a number of dominant themes that emerged from a close examination of experiencing within events of clinical practice. These key themes are briefly revisited in this chapter with a discussion of their significance for clinical and surgical training and medical education.

I have discussed in some detail that in the *thisness* of clinical practice, how surgeons make sense of their daily encounters in and of practice involves forms of *affective thinking*. This was best illustrated in the narrative accounts from Eleanor and Miranda in Chapter 8. Miranda described how caring for 'yet-to-die' patients had transformed the business of her daily ward round. She discussed the importance of finding time for these patients and their families because she concluded that 'they have the most questions' when confronted by a relative who is still alive despite being given a fatal prognosis.

Eleanor similarly described how an encounter with a child in pain reconfigured her attitude regarding how she responded to the demands exerted upon her as an on-call doctor. The analysis of both surgeons' encounters with the thisness of actual practice raises the following question: *what modes of thinking and being are important in cultivating an ability to cope with the immanence of surgical practice?* This is the central question that guided the examination of events of practice. It is answered in the four conclusions that are discussed in the following subsections.

The affective force of events of practice

Encounters with unfamiliar practice precipitate flows of affect which can creep up on us, overwhelming one with the intensity of the experience, triggering thoughts (what do I do here? how do I continue?), emotions (discomfort, unease, thrill, love, anger, fear) halting our ability to act or impelling us to move. This is the *affective force of events* of practice that emerges from any learning encounter or clinical event creating a difference for that individual – familiar ways of seeing and understanding the world are now ruptured and the resultant disparity urges one to find new ways that provide a resolution to this problematic of affect. In the example of Miranda, her modes of thinking and being, when confronted by termi-nally ill patients and their families, are precipitated by the state of affectations that emerge from this complex situation. She chooses to interact in specific ways with these patients and so resolves the tension that exists within herself and the chal-lenging situation she finds herself in. This form of affective response is implicated in her emerging subjectivity.

Thus, the affective force of encounters with unanticipated clinical practice can be experienced in ways that reflect how the encounter with practice comes to matter to her. This notion of mattering resonates with Gilbert Simondon's con-cept of invention. He asserts that invention is more than finding a solution to a problem. Instead, he emphasises it as the act of *establishing coherence* (Chabot 2003, p. 20), integrating incompatible elements to create a 'regime of functioning' (Massumi et al. 2009, p. 39) or a way of moving forward, that provides an answer to the initial disparity.

Form is immanent to clinical encounters of practice

The training materials and official documents of clinical practice anticipate a particular surgeon identity associated with specific skills. This was presented in Chapter 4 through the comparison of Official Care and Real Care. In the former, documents such as *Good Medical Practice* (2013) and *Good Surgical Practice* (2014) prescribe certain ways of being and acting that are framed as 'safe' and desirable attitudes and practices. These transcendent frameworks of practice are necessary to ensure that surgeons are trained with the critical skills that ensure competent and safe practice.

However, the reality of how a surgeon actually provides appropriate care in unexpected situations of clinical practice does not fit neatly into the prior categories of skill and practice. This is illustrated in the auto-ethnographic account of Chapter 5 describing the discovery of an 'errant testicle' in a hernia operation and in Mr. Martino's refusal to engage with his medical team in Chapter 3. The surgeons in these separate clinical episodes are forced by the *form* of the encounter – the ways in which the event of practice is prehended (taken account of) by the surgeon – to think and act in ways that are not necessarily subscribed to by the formal bodies of knowledge and practice.

The difference between providing *Official Care* and *Real Care* demonstrates how the immanent nature of clinical relations and practices is not captured by the hylomorphism of established modes of being and acting. The difficulty arises when surgeons are confronted by contingent events which have neither been described nor discussed by the official manuals of practice. These documents and ways of acting do not embrace the affective experiences that surround the *singular happenings* of putting approved skills into practice. This is exemplified by the 'speechlessness of practice' that characterises my experience at the organ procurement, an encounter in which I am unable to demonstrate the surgical skills that I have come to acquire. Such responses and reactions represent the local immanence of clinical events of practice.

How then are clinicians to be guided and supervised through the uncertainty of clinical events? I have argued using the theories of Whitehead, Deleuze and Simondon for a recognition of the intrinsic form that is immanent to all events of practice. That is, as an event of practice unfolds, the clinician prehends or takes account of the event by grasping the inherent form of the clinical encounter. The form of the encounter emerges through the relations that evolve and develop through processes of intra-action (Barad 2007) and interaction, creating complex layers of experiencing within the event of practice.

Therefore, in conceiving effective pedagogic strategies and practices, it is vital that trainers and educators consider how best to support learners as they grapple with prehending the form of events of practice. This struggle to grasp the event in a way that becomes meaningful to them either during the encounter or after it may exceed the resources of knowledge and skill that they are already familiar with (because it has been taught previously or experienced in the past). For surgical teachers this may constitute a contemplation of *the ways in which a trainer can draw alongside a learner* engaged in the thisness of practice, to attempt to 'see' and understand how the form of the learning encounter arises for them. Atkinson (2008, 2011) describes this principle as a 'pedagogy against the state': it resists the traditional practices that normalise learning encounters according to established categories of thinking and doing, otherwise regarded as transcendent values. This approach allows the learner and teacher to respond in ways that reflect what matters to them in the encounter and so embrace the *differences* that emerge from specific events of practice.

Power-knowledge: official training manuals and practice

In Chapters 4 and 5 I used Foucault's theory of power-knowledge (as well as insights from Butler and Bourdieu) to examine how training materials and policy documentation pedagogised the surgical trainee and trainer. I concluded, using the example of how a trainee's operative practice was scrutinised, that a learner's ability to operate is not viewed as an intrinsic capacity that can be discovered or developed, even though this may appear to be the objective of the technical teaching and assessment exercise. Instead, I suggested that the present paradigm of operative training constituted a particular discursive practice: it identified surgical skill in ways that inhibit or neglect to acknowledge other representations or signifiers of technical skill.

This becomes problematic within an educational and training context, if such a discursive practice occludes alternative signifiers of ability. The latter may constitute how operative practice *matters* to trainees and these forms of mattering may constitute personal forms of governance that modulate and influence how they learn.

This conclusion is not asserted to diminish the very important role that established foundational practices provide in training surgeons to operate competently and safely. Rather, what I advocate is an increased awareness of how curricular strategies can mould training practices to reflect exclusively, established components of skill which are considered critical to forming competence. The subjectivities of both trainee and trainer emerge from submitting (unknowingly) to the forms of power and governance inherent in this conception of operative practice and which also appear as obvious and natural processes.

An ethics of immanence

At the heart of this book is the finding of a necessary tension between an ethics of actual practice, contrasted with an ethics of transcendence. The former, I have contended, emerges from *real events of clinical practice*. In these encounters, a doctor has to make decisions in the 'here and now' according to the contingencies of the actual doctor-patient relations: *an immanent ethics of clinical practice*. An ethics of transcendence, refers to the forms of surgical care, set out in terms of clinical guidelines and ethical codes. Although they provide guidance for a doctor, they are not situated in actual events of practice and as such, I have argued, can be ineffective when confronted by problems in the 'here and now' of practice. In addition, I have shown that even when formal guidance is clear and applicable, surgeons may not follow the approved practices due to various 'barriers' (personal beliefs, the conflicting demands of busy practice) that preclude this. This was demonstrated in Chapter 5 in the tale of the unusual hernia operation and in Chapter 8 in Eleanor's second account of a woman in pain.

To explore how surgeons actualise practice and to theorise on how the structurisation of medical practice can enable and also control actualisations of surgical practice, I applied Gilles Deleuze's theories. Deleuze proposes that *real learning* (Atkinson 2008) is a process in which a subject expands on their capacities through an engagement with ways of thinking, being and doing that are yet to emerge and become concrete ('potentialities'). This echoes my earlier point that surgical and medical pedagogies must include strategies that allow a teacher to 'draw alongside' a learner. Such an approach complements the teaching of important foundational knowledge and skills as well as enhancing local flows of learning that can extend, enable and strengthen a learner in practice.

Deleuze advocates a conception of ethics as a set of facultative rules that 'evaluate what we do according to the immanent mode of existence that it implies' (Smith 2012, p. 176). This theory of ethics exceeds moral concerns and instead precipitates the following questions: what *can* I do, what am I *capable* of doing? rather than what *must* I do? (which refers to issues of morality). Therefore, the mode of being is determined through a subject's power to act in an encounter (which is influenced by affective relations), or otherwise through the inability of the subject to act to their fullest capacity.

A surgical pedagogy grounded in an onto-ethics of immanence is a paradigm of learning and teaching in clinical environments that is premised on notions of *becoming* (individuation) and *difference* (new ways to understand, make sense, act etc.) within local flows of events of practice. It promotes an ethics of practice which encompasses transcendent frameworks of how doctors should and shouldn't behave (as prescribed in guidelines), and then proceeds to exceed these confines. This is not to devalue the assimilated values and practices of surgery but to draw attention to how they may be limited in dealing fully with the complexities of actual clinical practice.

An ethics of immanence recognises the ideas, actions and subjects that emerge from the dynamic flows of local experiences of practice. Put another way, an immanent ethics of surgical practice is grounded in the *thisness* or 'here and now' of an encounter of clinical practice: it may trigger the following question, what does it mean to provide care for this patient? Such a response is consistent with the nature of entangled practices and subjectivities that constitute the worlds of surgical practice and which I have sought to illustrate in the arguments presented in this book.

9.3   Modes of mattering and becoming: the wider implications of my research findings

I stated in the first chapter that this book is concerned with articulating the emotional dimensions of practice and in particular how events of clinical practice come to *matter* to learners and practitioners. Through a process of mattering, events of practice make sense and become meaningful for the individual practitioner. As such, encounters with clinical practice can have the effect of producing ontological and epistemological growth. Modes of becoming and modes of being (ethics) emerge from an engagement with clinical events of practice. The question arises, therefore, as to how to create clinical pedagogies that are sensitive to the different modes of mattering? How can surgical practices inherit the specific modes of mattering of the entities that constitute daily encounters in practice?

Surgery is distinguished as a craft specialty characterised by 'doing' in response to what is seen, felt and anticipated. It is a discipline that relies on visual and tactile stimuli to provide information to the surgeon both in operative and non-operative (clinics, wards) environments. The potent odours, the graphic and acute images of flesh and viscera, the differing textures and vivid colours of tissues all combine to elicit strong sensations and responses. These experiences constitute a whole world of affects and senses which the trainee can also encounter as a sense of apprehension. I suggest that these entities, the affective responses they spark and the intra actions that form and develop between them, come together in a *dynamic mode of becoming* which constructs the patient-doctor relation in an event of practice.

The paradoxical challenge to surgical practice is to resist thinking about these entities as detached, discrete components of experience but at the same time being careful to consider their independent and differential modes of existence. Therefore, clinical practices must develop ways of responding to the dynamic problem of different modes of mattering that can coexist in a clinical encounter and which compose the becoming of an event of practice. The onto-ethical concern that arises from these processes of mattering is how to respond in the here-and-now in ways that attend to the obligations posed by the constituent parts of the encounter. An example is the 'problematic existence' of Mr. Cunningham, the transplant recipient I describe at the beginning of this chapter, whom I operated on. In the environment of the operating theatre, his 'stubborn' existence as a human being with past experiences and a life story are reduced (unavoidably) to the medical parameters that constitute his being as a patient. I as a surgeon am compelled to view him through this medical lens of disease – this is how I am obligated in this clinical environment.

I advocate an approach to clinical practice that is first concerned with recognizing and understanding the *various modes of mattering* that develop and form within an event of practice. Second, a consideration of how the differential modes of mattering determine how the patient's mode of being is recognised and valued in the clinical situation so that he is captured beyond the medical parameters of his clinical status. This is the challenge of an immanent ethics of clinical practice – how the surgeon becomes 'response-able' (Harraway 2008, p. 88) in relation to a complex of entities (Whatmore, 1997) that compose the clinical encounter.

9.4   Final thoughts

I have discussed and argued the need for a surgical education that exceeds the traditions of the original craft of surgery. I advocate for pedagogies of surgical training and clinical education that are liberated from the tyranny of competency-based training and meticulous assessments. The latter are necessary to develop a system of medical training that is accountable and transparent. Its purpose is to assure the competence and professionalism of doctors, thereby ensuring that patients receive the best care and their welfare is prioritised.

However, I propose an educational project that remains sensitive to these existing concerns but reconfigures learning as a responsiveness to the haecceities of practice. In this conception of learning, surgical training is grounded in a metaphysics of immanence and becoming. This would create an alternate yet complementary epistemology of clinical practice, one that is concerned with exploring how to cultivate connections between the mode of mattering of an entity and the mode of responding of the practice. In surgical practice this is best illustrated by the affectations triggered within a clinical encounter: first, how the encounter with practice affects a surgeon in terms of how she is obligated by the human and non-human actants in the encounter, and, second, how the encounter itself is affected by the surgeon's obligatory positions.

Employing an epistemology of practice through an ethics of response-ability is a way of being accountable for what emerges from the uncertainty of clinical practice. This may prove an enduring strategy in professional practice, in which the proliferation of mandatory regulation and the dominance of the standards discourse have not been as effective as was first anticipated in preparing professional for the complexities of real practice.

References

Atkinson, D. (2008). "Pedagogy Against the State." *International Journal of Art and Design Education*, 27 (3): 226–240.

Atkinson, D. (2011). *Art, Equality and Learning: Pedagogies Against the State*. Rotterdam, Boston and Taipei: Sense Publishers.

Badiou, A. (2005). *Being and Event*. London and New York: Continuum.

Barad, K. (2007). *Meeting the Universe Halfway: Quantum Physics and the Entanglement of Matter and Meaning*. Duke University Press.

Chabot, P. (2003). *The Philosophy of Simondon*, trans. Krefetz, A., and Kirkpatrick, G. Bloomsbury Academic.

General Medical Council. (2013). *Good Medical Practice*. London: General Medical Council.

Harraway, D. J. (2008). *When Species Meet*. University of Minnesotta.

Massumi, B., De Boever, A., et al. (2009). "'Technical Mentality' Revisited: Brian Massumi on Gilbert Simondon." *Parrhesia*, 7: 36–45. Retrieved from www.parrhesiajournal.org/parrhesia07/parrhesia07_massumi.pdf.

Royal College of Surgeons of England. (2014). *Good Surgical Practice*. RCSE: Professional Standards.

Smith, D. W. (2012). *Essays on Deleuze*. Edinburgh University Press.

Whatmore, S. (1997). "Dissecting the Autonomous Self: Hybrid Cartographies for a Relational Ethics." *Environment and Planning D: Society and Space*, 15: 37–53.

Index